patrick
HOLFORD

SAY
NO TO
ARTHRITIS

THE PROVEN DRUG-FREE
GUIDE TO PREVENTING
AND RELIEVING
ARTHRITIS

piatkus

PIATKUS

First published in Great Britain in 1999 by Piatkus Books
This updated and expanded version first published 2009

Reprinted 2009

A CIP catalogue record for this book
is available from the British Library

ISBN 978-0-7499-2013-5

Typeset in Bembo by Phoenix Photosetting, Chatham, Kent
Printed and bound in the UK by CPI Mackays, Chatham ME5 8TD

Papers used by Piatkus are natural, renewable and recyclable
products sourced from well-managed forests and certified
in accordance with the rules of the Forest Stewardship Council.

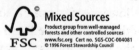

Mixed Sources
Product group from well-managed
forests and other controlled sources
www.fsc.org Cert no. SGS-COC-004081
FSC © 1996 Forest Stewardship Council

Piatkus
An imprint of
Little, Brown Book Group
100 Victoria Embankment
London EC4Y 0DY

An Hachette UK Company
www.hachette.co.uk

www.piatkus.co.uk

ABOUT THE AUTHOR

Patrick Holford BSc, DipION, FBANT is a leading spokesman on nutrition in the media, specialising in the field of mental health. He is author of 30 books, translated into over 20 languages and selling over a million copies worldwide, including the *Optimum Nutrition Bible* and *Optimum Nutrition for the Mind*.

Patrick Holford started his academic career in the field of psychology. In 1984 he founded the Institute for Optimum Nutrition (ION), an independent educational charity, and was involved in groundbreaking research showing that multi-vitamins can increase children's IQ scores – research that was published in the *Lancet* and the subject of a *Horizon* documentary in the 1980s. He was one of the first promoters of the importance of zinc, antioxidants, essential fats, low-GL diets and homocysteine-lowering B vitamins such as folic acid.

He is director of the Food for the Brain Foundation and the Brain Bio Centre, the Foundation's treatment centre. He is an honorary fellow of the British Association of Nutritional Therapy, as well as a member of the Nutrition Therapy Council.

CONTENTS

ACKNOWLEDGEMENTS

This book would not have been possible without the help and support of many people. I am especially indebted to Liz Efiong for her help researching and editing this new edition, and to Natalie Savona for her help with editing and researching the original book. Also to Michael Ash, osteopath, naturopath and nutritional therapist, for his material on fibromyalgia in Chapter 18, Clive Lathey, osteopath, for his help with exercise for reducing back pain in Chapter 24, and to Joe Sharpe for the osteoporosis exercises in Chapter 17.

GUIDE TO ABBREVIATIONS AND MEASURES

1 gram (g) = 1,000 milligrams (mg) = 1,000,000 micrograms (mcg or µg)
Most vitamins are measured in milligrams or micrograms. Vitamins A, D and E are also measured in International Units (iu), a measurement designed to standardise the various forms of these vitamins that have different potencies.
1mcg of retinol (1mcg RE) = 3.3iu of vitamin A
1mcg RE of beta-carotene = 6mcg of beta-carotene
100iu of vitamin D = 2.5mcg
100iu of vitamin E = 67mg
1 pound (lb) = 16 ounces (oz)   2.2lb = 1 kilogram (kg)
1 pint = 0.6 litres   1.76 pints = 1 litre
In this book, calories means kilocalories (kcals)
2 teaspoons (tsp) = 1 dessertspoon (dsp)
3 teaspoons (tsp) = 1 tablespoon (tbsp)
1.5 dessertspoons = 1 tablespoon (tbsp)

REFERENCES AND
FURTHER SOURCES OF
INFORMATION

Numerous references from respected scientific literature have been used in writing this book. Details of specific studies referred to are listed on pages 316–42. More details on most of these studies can be found on the Internet for those wishing to dig deeper. On page 343, you will find a list of the best books to read to follow up or understand more about this subject.

DISCLAIMER

Although all the nutrients and dietary changes referred to in this book have been proven safe, those seeking help for specific medical conditions are advised to consult a qualified nutritional therapist, doctor or equivalent health professional. If you are taking medication, I recommend you check with your doctor if there are any contraindications between the medication you are on and the supplements you wish to take. The recommendations given in this book are solely intended as education and information, and should not be taken as medical advice. Neither the authors nor the publisher accept liability for readers who choose to self-prescribe.

**All supplements should be kept out of the reach of
infants and young children.**

HOW TO USE THIS BOOK

Arthritis is not a single disease. There are many different kinds of arthritis, as well as associated conditions that are not technically classified as arthritis, such as osteoporosis, fibromyalgia and polymyalgia. This book aims to give you clear guidance on natural approaches to all kinds of arthritis and such associated conditions.

Part 1 helps you identify what kind of condition you have. It also introduces you to some basic information (for example, what joints are made of, how healthy joints work, what inflammation is, how it causes pain and how arthritis progresses), giving you a clearer understanding of the basis behind different approaches to the treatment of arthritis. It will help you identify the possible risk factors that can contribute to the development of arthritis.

Part 2 covers nine nutritional approaches to switching off inflammation, and hence reducing pain naturally, by dealing with many of the true underlying factors that lead you to suffer from arthritis.

Part 3 Once inflammation has been switched off, the next stage in recovery is to rebuild healthy joints, which is the subject of this part. Yes, you can rebuild your joints.

Part 4 focuses on related conditions: osteoporosis, fibromyalgia and gout.

Part 5 tells you what you actually need to do to help your body heal itself – the practical measures, not the theory. So, if you've had enough of theory and research, you can turn straight to Part 5 and get on with it!

At the end of the more complicated chapters you will find a useful summary, if you prefer to dip into the book.

A few words of caution:

1 Never stop or change medication prescribed by your doctor without his or her knowledge and consent. However, you will probably find that your need for painkillers naturally reduces.
2 Do not exceed the doses of vitamins, minerals or amino acids recommended in this book.
3 It's best to carry out these recommendations under the guidance of a nutritional therapist. My website will help you how to find one in your area (see www.patrick holford.com).
4 If you experience adverse reactions to any of these nutrients, stop taking the supplement you suspect is causing the reaction. If the symptoms persist, see your doctor or a nutritional therapist.

Although all the recommendations made in this book are based on proper research, and involve substances with minimal or no known risk of adverse reactions, the author cannot be responsible for the outcome of your choosing to experiment with these recommendations.

INTRODUCTION

According to Dr Robert Bingham, a specialist in the treatment of arthritis, 'No person who is in good nutritional health develops rheumatoid or osteoarthritis.' Yet, by the age of 60, nine in every ten people in the UK have arthritis. According to the Arthritis Research Campaign, nearly 9 million adults in the UK (that's 19 per cent of the adult population) have seen their GP in the last year for arthritis or a related condition, and 45 per cent experience symptoms. For all sufferers, arthritis means living with pain and stiffness. For some, it is a living hell and can be life-threatening. Yet arthritis is not an inevitable consequence of ageing. Arthritis can be prevented and the underlying causes can be eliminated. This book tells you how to:

- Reduce pain and inflammation without drugs.
- Identify and eliminate the causes of arthritis.
- Recover and gain mobility.
- Prevent arthritis and stop it progressing.
- Prevent osteoporosis and improve your bone density.
- Reduce muscle pain and prevent fibromyalgia.

WHY SUFFER?

Some time ago I had a call from a client I hadn't seen in several years. 'What you recommended sorted out my arthritis, but now the symptoms are beginning to return again,' she told me. A simple diet and some supplements, based on a new way of looking at arthritis, kept her pain-free for seven more years. Around that time a woman in her seventies came to see me. She had marked degeneration of her lower spine and had considerable persistent pain in her back and left leg. I didn't expect to be able to do much, but I put her on an appropriate diet plus supplements. Six weeks later she returned to report that she no longer had pain in her leg, and her back pain had decreased by half. Ten years on she remains free of pain.

Later on I'll tell you about Ed, who suffered from constant knee pain. Despite having seen all the top specialists and tried all the conventional and quite a few alternative approaches, nothing changed. 'Since following your advice my discomfort has decreased 95 to 100 per cent,' said Ed, three months later.

Why do so few people recover? And why do one in ten people never develop arthritis in the first place? In some communities, nine people in ten never develop arthritis.

Arthritis means inflammation (*itis*) of a joint (*arthron*). It's a term I use loosely here to describe a whole host of problems affecting joints, bones and muscles, but it's not simply an unavoidable 'wear and tear' degenerative disease. For example, in some African communities, where people spend hours every day walking without shoes, arthritis is exceedingly rare.

Your body is the very latest model, shaped over millions of years of evolution, designed to deliver decades of good service. Why, therefore, should you accept that when a part starts misbehaving there is nothing you can do except dull the pain?

Arthritis starts with joint aches and pains. Many people put up with these early warning signs until they develop into something a little more persistent. Then, a visit to the doctor may result in a prescription for an anti-inflammatory or painkilling drug. Conventional drug treatments do nothing to cure the disease. At best they reduce the pain. At worst, they speed up the progress of the disease. Severe arthritis is probably responsible for more suffering than any other disease, including both cancer and heart disease. That's the bad news.

The good news is that there is an alternative approach. Arthritis can be prevented and the underlying causes can be eliminated. If you stop the disease early enough you can hope for a complete recovery. If your arthritis has already resulted in considerable damage to your joints you may, at best, be able to halt the progress of the disease and reduce the pain with little or no recourse to drugs. Either way, to find the best approach to treating your arthritis, you need to identify the likely factors that contributed to its original development, which is what Part 1 addresses.

THINKING DIFFERENTLY

The true solution requires you to think differently. As Albert Einstein said, 'The problems we have created cannot be solved at the same level of thinking we were at when we created them.' The core philosophy of a nutrition-based approach is the understanding that arthritis results when core underlying biological systems can't cope any more. It's called a 'systems-based' approach, because I'll be exploring fundamental body systems, such as your hormonal balance, blood sugar balance, detoxification and inflammatory control processes, which normally keep everything working in your body. And I'll be talking about a few you might never have heard of; for example, methylation. The key question I'll be exploring with you again and again is: what makes your body tip into a new state in which your joints hurt and degenerate?

By now you've probably realised that there is no magic bullet; each drug that has promised one to users has ended up shooting them in the foot. Instead, you'll discover that you have to change, or rather support, these key underlying biological processes, which are entirely dependent on nutrition, because we are literally made from, and run on, nutrients. It is fundamental.

In this 'systems-based' way of thinking it's important to understand that what you need to restore your body and joints to a new state (free of pain and no longer degenerating) is a set of circumstances that is far more extreme than those needed to maintain it in its present state. You have to 'tip' your system back to health. Simply changing your diet won't do this, although it might provide a little relief. What you need to do is provide your body with the right diet that's free of the foods that might aggravate it, and provide the exact nutrients and natural painkillers that will help to restore normal pain-free function and heal the joints. In practical terms this means taking specific supplements – not for ever, although some are worth taking long term, but certainly until you achieve significant relief.

UNDERSTANDING THE RESEARCH

In the chapters that follow I will refer to many research trials carried out to investigate different possible causes of arthritis and approaches to its treatment. I have tended to avoid anecdotal reports of arthritis cures, except to illustrate a proven approach or to highlight a potential area for more research.

The best studies are controlled, 'double-blind trials' with objective and subjective measures of improvement. For example, increased flexibility of a joint that has been objectively measured, together with a decrease in the erythrocyte sedimentation rate (ESR) in the blood (which indicates inflammation), both provide strong evidence that something has really happened. If backed up by subjective improvement – in other words, if the patient feels better – this is even more positive, since that is, after all, what treatment sets out to do. However, it is important to know if the actual disease process is being arrested or if it is simply the pain that is being masked.

Controlled studies involve comparisons between two similar groups of people: one receiving the treatment in question, the other not. Sometimes both groups remain on painkillers, but the 'experimental' group also takes a nutritional supplement. This tells us whether a supplement plus painkillers is more effective than painkillers alone. However, the effect could be in the mind of the person if they knew they were taking vitamins. Some researchers use patients as their own control by monitoring them without treatment, then administering treatment and recording the difference. But, you also have to take into account whether the disease would have got worse or better on its own anyway.

For this reason scientists love 'double-blind' trials. This means that each group of people is given, for example, either a supplement, or a dummy ('placebo') supplement. Neither the person nor the experimenter knows which is which until the trial is over. The difference between the results in one group and the other cannot, therefore, be caused by a psychological effect or by bias on the part of the experimenter. As good as these trials are, however, they have limitations. For example, how do you test a diet in this way? You cannot give someone a placebo diet. Also, the problem with sole reliance on randomised placebo controlled trials (called RCTs) is that they test only one piece of the jigsaw. In every case of arthritis recovery that I've heard of, the person has combined a number of critical pieces of the jigsaw. I'd like you to know all the evidence – and there is a lot. That's the science.

The art of recovery is in knowing how to put the correct pieces together. I'm going to identify which pieces are likely to make the biggest difference for you, and, in Part 5, show you how to put them together into your strategy and action plan for reversing arthritis.

Wishing you the best of pain-free and drug-free health.

Patrick Holford

PART 1

UNDERSTANDING ARTHRITIS

CHAPTER 1

....

GETTING THE RIGHT DIAGNOSIS

There are two major kinds of arthritis, and many, less common, arthritis-like conditions. The most common kind is osteoarthritis (sometimes called OA). This 'wear and tear' disease affects joints that have been injured or simply worn out, often through poor posture and/or lack of mobility, which is necessary to keep joints flexible and healthy. This is much more common in people over the age of 50. Rheumatoid arthritis (sometimes called RA), however, is less common and more complex, but can strike at any age – even in childhood. It affects younger people and is 'systemic', meaning that the whole body's immune system and inflammatory responses go into overdrive, perhaps nudged by hereditary factors and infections, as well as by diet and lifestyle.

OSTEOARTHRITIS

About 80 per cent of people over the age of 50 show osteoarthritis-like joint damage, and a quarter of them experience pain. By the age of 60, over 90 per cent of people show evidence on X-ray of arthritis-like joint damage. Whereas osteoarthritis occurs later in life, painful and stiff knee problems – often diagnosed as chondromalacia (an abnormal softening or degeneration of joint cartilage, especially of the knee) – occur frequently in people under 40.

Under the age of 45, osteoarthritis is more common in men; over the age of 45, it's more common in women, probably due to reduced calcium absorption after the menopause. It starts as stiffness, usually of the weight-bearing joints such as the knees, hips and back, and progresses to pain on movement. The joints then become increasingly swollen and inflexible.

Osteoarthritis is marked by a loss of cartilage, which leads to excess friction and overuse. (Figure 1 shows a healthy joint with its cartilage.) This, in turn, leads to drying out of the cartilage and further loss of cartilage. Eventually collagen, the protein matrix of bone, starts to break down in the ends of the

A healthy joint consists of bone covered by a layer of smooth, less brittle cartilage and separated from the opposite bone by a lubricating synovial fluid kept within a synovial membrane sac.

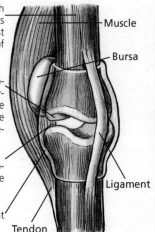

Bone consists of collagen (a kind of protein), together with proteoglycans, which bind in the minerals calcium, phosphorus and magnesium. Calcium is the greatest single constituent of bone – 99 per cent of the body's calcium is found within bone.

Cartilage consists of collagen and proteoglycans made from protein and carbohydrate. Cartilage is smooth and less brittle than bone, thereby protecting the bone ends and maintaining smooth joint movements.

Synovial fluid is a lubricating liquid produced in synovial cells and secreted into the joint space to lubricate the joint.

Synovial membrane surrounds the joint space, enclosing the synovial fluid.

Figure 1 – A healthy joint

bones. This leads to a thickening of bone ends and the formation of osteophytes (large bone spurs), often making the joint appear enlarged. Synovial fluid becomes stickier and less able to lubricate; the whole joint area becomes inflamed; and movement is increasingly restricted. Calcium, instead of being incorporated into bone, may get dumped in other tissues of the body, such as muscle, leading to muscle pain and stiffness.

Osteoarthritis is usually triggered by 'wear and tear' (for example, bad posture), inadequate diet, a trauma such as a strain, obesity, or another disease. The major causes are thought to be improper diet and certain lifestyle factors, which, over the years, can upset the body's metabolism and ability to keep joints healthy. The progression of osteoarthritis suggests that the body is trying to heal damaged tissue within the joint.

When there is evidence of joint damage, but no pain or inflammation, the condition is called arthrosis.

RHEUMATOID ARTHRITIS

There are an estimated half a million people in the UK, and 3 million in the US, who suffer with rheumatoid arthritis, and around 80 per cent of them are women. Although the peak age is between 30 and 50, many people develop rheumatoid arthritis in childhood! Unlike osteoarthritis, this condition often affects the whole body, and usually both sides of the body (for example, both wrists, rather than simply a weight-bearing joint). It most often affects fingers, wrists, knees and ankles but can also affect other parts of the body such as heart tissue and muscles.

Rheumatoid arthritis starts with inflammation of the synovial membrane. Consequently the joint becomes inflamed and enlarged, causing pain, swelling, stiffness, and loss of function in the joints and possibly other parts of the body. The synovial membrane actually produces chemicals that further irritate the joint and start a process of degeneration in the

1 A healthy joint consists of strong bones, which are essentially minerals in a collagen (protein) matrix. Cartilage on the edge of bones is protected from the opposing bone and cartilage by a sac containing synovial fluid, which effectively lubricates the joint.

2 Cartilage is made from proteoglycans and collagen. Overuse and dietary imbalances can lead to a breakdown of cartilage. Synovial fluid becomes less lubricating. The loss of cartilage also leads to a breakdown of collagen components and weakening of bone. Bone ends become uneven and osteophytes (large bone spurs) form. Inflammation restricts movement.

3 Loss of calcium balance can lead to calcium being dumped in soft tissues, causing muscle pain. Bone ends can become fused together. The progressive stages of arthritis suggest that the body is trying to heal damaged tissue. The goal is to enable the body to rebuild its collagen matrix and restore healthy bones, cartilage and synovial membranes.

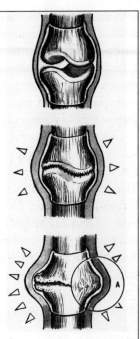

Figure 2 – How arthritis develops

cartilage and ultimately the bone. Rheumatoid joints are often warm, and sufferers may have a slight fever. They are likely to feel tired and generally run down.

The cause of this form of arthritis is more mysterious, but it may be due to immune system problems, perhaps triggered by a viral or bacterial infection, or a genetic weakness (it is thought that rheumatoid arthritis is, in part, hereditary). Rheumatoid arthritis often starts and flares up when nutrition is under par, probably because good nutrition is vital for immune strength. Most rheumatoid arthritis sufferers develop antibodies that attack normal components of the body, as if the immune system has malfunctioned. This is why rheumatoid arthritis is called an autoimmune condition – there is evidence that the body's own immune system attacks the joints. Rheumatoid arthritis can be mild, or severe and active most of the time, last for many years, and lead to serious joint damage and disability. It is so disabling that half of all patients have to stop working within ten years of diagnosis.

ANKYLOSING SPONDYLITIS

The condition ankylosing spondylitis differs from other arthritic conditions in that it starts with inflammation of the ends of the ligaments, where they attach to the bones. This most commonly starts in the sacroiliac joint, where the pelvis and spine meet. As the disease progresses, the vertebrae at the base of the spine start to fuse together. The symptoms are lower back pain and stiffness. As the area becomes more and more inflamed, joint pain and stiffness may also occur in other parts of the body.

When there is evidence of spinal fusion, but no pain or inflammation, the condition is called spondylosis.

GOUT

One in every 200 people will suffer from gout. It is caused by a build-up of uric acid, a substance in the blood that should be excreted from the body via the kidneys. Excess uric acid can form crystals that lodge in joints and tissue, most commonly the big toe, causing localised pain. When gout is present there is usually increased inflammation, which may affect other joints.

OSTEOPOROSIS

The condition osteoporosis is the gradual loss of bone density. As such it is not specifically a disease of the joints, but of the bones themselves. However, the health of bones does affect joints, and many underlying mechanisms that are now thought to contribute to osteoporosis are shared with osteoarthritis.

Osteoporosis is thought to affect over two million people in the UK. It occurs twice as commonly in women, and is most prevalent in women after the menopause. One in three women and one in 12 men have a fracture as a result of osteoporosis by the age of 70. It is usually identified only when a fracture occurs – often of the hip – and it is therefore considered a hidden epidemic. Forty people die every day as a result of fractures caused by osteoporosis.

Loss of bone density occurs because calcium is not being properly deposited in bone, or is actively being removed. Many factors are known to upset the calcium balance in bone. These include excess protein consumption, excess tea, coffee or alcohol, blood sugar problems, thyroid or parathyroid hormone imbalances, stress, loss of oestrogen and progesterone in the menopausal years, lack of weight-bearing exercise, lack of magnesium, and lack of vitamin D or sunlight. These factors are covered in more detail in Part 3, and Chapter 17 gives you a strategy for preventing and reversing osteoporosis.

POLYMYALGIA AND FIBROMYALGIA

An increasingly common problem, polymyalgia mainly affects older women, in which muscles (rather than joints) become stiff and painful. The onset is usually rapid and suggests that the problem may be triggered by a virus or by accumulated stress – 'the straw that breaks the camel's back' – thus initiating a rheumatoid-like condition, marked by inflammation. The recommendations given in this book for reducing inflammation without drugs are often helpful (see Part 2).

Another debilitating condition causing muscle aches, pain and stiffness is fibromyalgia. This is different from polymyalgia in that it is not characterised by inflammation. The pain is thought to be caused by problems with energy production within cells, leading to muscle tension. These conditions are discussed fully in Chapter 18.

OSTEOMALACIA OR RICKETS

The disease osteomalacia (in adults), or rickets (in children), is caused by a deficiency in vitamin D. We need this vitamin in order to use calcium properly. A lack of it leads to weak and pliable bones, resulting in bone deformities such as bow legs or bent fingers and toes. Vitamin D is made in the skin in the presence of sunlight, so both diet and exposure of the skin to the sun play a part. People with dark skin, who get little direct exposure to sunlight, and who also eat a vegan diet (without eggs, dairy products, meat or fish), are most at risk.

DISPLACED INTERVERTEBRAL DISC

Often wrongly referred to as a 'slipped disc', displaced inter-vertebral disc occurs when two vertebrae in the spine are out of alignment. This can put pressure on the spinal nerve that runs through the spinal column. Poor spinal alignment can also lead to rupture of the synovial sac between vertebrae, causing tremendous pain both from inflammation and through nerve compression. Eventually the vertebrae can fuse together.

BURSITIS, TENDONITIS AND TENOSYNOVITIS

These three inflammatory conditions do not affect joints as such. Bursitis refers to inflammation of the fluid-filled cush-ions that separate muscle from bone. The most common sites are in the shoulders, elbows and knees. Tendonitis is inflam-mation where the tendons attach to bone, and tenosynovitis is inflammation of the sheath surrounding the tendon.

Terms such as lumbago (back ache) and rheumatism (systemic joint and muscle ache) usually refer to symptoms that can be described more accurately by one of the above types of arthritic condition.

CHAPTER 2

······················

WHY ARTHRITIS?

When you get ill, two questions usually come to mind. The first is: 'How do I get better?' And the second is: 'Why did I get ill in the first place?' Knowing why you have developed a disease doesn't cure it, but it is usually the first step towards finding a solution. In the search for the cause of arthritis, many factors have been considered, including diet,

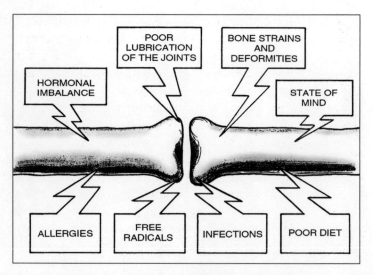

Figure 3 – Factors that affect the bones

physical exercise, posture, climate, hormones, infections, allergies, genetics, old age and stress. Most of these have proven relevant to at least some arthritis sufferers. But what is the cause? I believe the answer – as for most diseases – is that arthritis does not have a single cause. The symptoms of arthritis, or of any arthritis-like disease, are the result of an accumulation of factors: accumulated stresses eventually reach a tipping point and trigger inflammation, causing joint, bone and muscle degeneration.

The likely factors that contribute to the development of this painful condition are:

Poor lubrication of the joints Good nutrition is needed to make sure the synovial fluid between joints stays fluid and lubricating. Cartilage and synovial fluid contain proteoglycans, which can be provided by certain foods. That's where nutrients such as glucosamine are beneficial – I'll explain exactly how in Chapter 16.

Hormonal imbalance Hormones control calcium balance in the body. If the body's hormones are out of control, bones and joints can become porous and subject to wear and tear. Calcium can then be deposited in the wrong place, resulting in arthritic 'spurs'. The problem is not usually insufficient calcium intake, but rather the loss of calcium balance in the body. Vitamin D, which is actually a hormone, is vital in this regard.

A lack of exercise, too much tea, coffee, alcohol or chocolate, exposure to toxic metals like lead, excessive stress or underlying blood sugar or thyroid imbalances all upset calcium control. This can be worse after the menopause, probably due to the loss of oestrogen and progesterone. However, oestrogen dominance – in other words, too much oestrogen relative to progesterone – also makes arthritis worse. It's all a question of balance. Another hormone, insulin, stimulates the synthesis of proteoglycans, from which cartilage is made.[1] In

Chapter 7 I'll explain the link between blood sugar problems, insulin resistance and arthritis. Also, people with underactive thyroid glands are more likely to suffer from arthritis.

Allergies and sensitivities Almost everyone who suffers from rheumatoid arthritis, and many who suffer from osteoarthritis, have food and/or chemical allergies or sensitivities that make their symptoms flare up. Some allergies cause arthritis in the first place. Others develop as a consequence of medication, inducing gut damage that makes matters worse. The most common food allergies are to wheat and dairy produce. It's well worth avoiding these foods strictly for one month to see whether this reduces the problem. You'll find more on this in Chapter 9.

Free radicals In all inflamed joints, a battle is taking place in which the body is trying to deal with the damage. Some of the key weapons of war faced by the body are free oxidising radicals (or free radicals, for short). These are like the body's own nuclear waste, made from oxygen reacting with glucose, the end result of breathing and eating. The reaction releases energy that allows our cells to work, but it also creates dangerous oxygen by-products, which can destroy cells and damage body tissue. Some free radicals are made through normal body processes. Eating a lot of fried food, for example, or smoking cigarettes, will increase them.

The body protects itself from free radicals with an army of antioxidant nutrients, such as vitamins A, C and E, and antioxidant enzymes, which contain minerals such as zinc and selenium. Specific foods, ranging from oregano to cherries, are especially high in antioxidants. I'll show you which foods to eat more of so that you can increase your antioxidant potential in Chapter 10.

The body even generates free radicals to destroy misbehaving cells such as cancer cells or invaders such as viruses. If the immune system isn't working properly, as in rheumatoid arthritis, it produces too many free radicals, which can damage the tissue around the joint. A low intake of antioxidant nutrients can therefore make arthritis worse.

Infections Any infection, be it viral or bacterial, weakens the immune system, which controls inflammation. But some viruses and bacteria particularly affect the joints by lodging in them and recurring when your immune defences are low. Often the immune system can harm surrounding tissue in its efforts to fight an infection, like an army which lays its own country waste when trying to get rid of an invader. Building up your immune defences through optimum nutrition is the natural solution.

Bone strain and deformities Any damage or strain, often caused by faulty posture, increases the risk of developing arthritis. A yearly check-up with an osteopath or chiropractor, plus regular exercise to increase joint suppleness and strength is the best prevention. Once arthritis has set in, special exercises can help to reduce pain and stiffness.

State of mind There is little question that arthritis, particularly rheumatoid arthritis, can create major stress both for the sufferer and their family.[2] But to what extent does psychology encourage the physical changes that lead to arthritis?

As long ago as 1936, the onset of rheumatoid arthritis was associated with factors such as marital problems, work-related stress and worry.[3] More recently, research at the University of Maryland School of Medicine has shown that an eight-week meditation training programme, followed by a four-month maintenance programme, significantly reduced psychological distress and improved general wellbeing in rheumatoid arthritis patients.[4]

While Dr Ronald Lamont-Havers was national medical director of the Arthritis and Rheumatism Foundation he examined hundreds of prison inmates and found only a negligible incidence of rheumatoid arthritis. In his opinion, 'These individuals who let out their angers and aggressive feelings so violently that they wound up behind bars had practically no RA. Emotional stress, brought on by hidden anger, fear or worry, often accompanies the beginning of arthritis.'[5]

The mind–body connection

Many ancient philosophies, and most modern theories of psychology, consider the mind and body to be intimately connected. Imbalances in a particular system in the body are thought to correspond with mental and emotional imbalances that may seek expression through the physical body. The musculoskeletal system is considered to be the physical manifestation of a person's need for space, authority and ownership. So, according to this theory, a person who has been denied their own space and authority in the world may be more prone to musculoskeletal problems. We use the phrase 'spineless' to mean someone who doesn't stand up for themselves.

Chronic arthritis is itself a great stress.[6] It is sadly no surprise that a large proportion of people with rheumatoid arthritis have been found to also suffer from depression, marital difficulties and low self-esteem. One key factor is the thought of having a disease of unknown outcome, with no knowledge of a treatment that really works. This leads to the belief that effective solutions are not available to control or eliminate either the disease or other life stresses.

Yet, as you will discover from this book, unless you have already exhausted all the nutritional approaches to arthritis, there is much you can do to improve the outcome of any form of the disease, without the risk of side effects. And there are always ways of dealing with pressures and difficult situations.

Chapter 12 gives some simple and practical tips for coping with life's stresses.

Poor diet Most people with arthritis have a history of poor diet, which paves the way for many of the above risk factors. Too much refined carbohydrate and sugar, too much of the wrong kind of fat and not enough essential fats, too much protein and too many stimulants (coffee, tea, alcohol, cigarettes) can all exacerbate arthritic problems. A lack of any of a number of vital vitamins, minerals and essential fats could, in itself, precipitate joint problems. As I mentioned in the Introduction, according to Dr Robert Bingham, a specialist in the treatment of arthritis, 'No person who is in good nutritional health develops rheumatoid or osteoarthritis.'

Great results can be achieved with arthritis by taking all these factors into account: eliminating possible risks, improving lifestyle, and following an optimal diet and supplement programme based on your individual needs. Pain and inflammation can be reduced, mobility can be increased, and, although it doesn't happen overnight, there is clear evidence that damaged joints can heal. All these factors are discussed in more detail later in this book.

CHAPTER 3

HOW YOUR BODY MAKES PAIN

The first indication that you may be developing arthritis is joint pain. Pain and inflammation are the body's way of saying, 'Help!' Although it is important to understand and deal with the underlying causes, taking painkillers and anti-inflammatory substances can help to calm down excessive and harmful inflammation, taking the body out of 'emergency' mode. Drugs can reduce pain by blocking chemicals that trigger inflammation, but they don't come without side effects, which is why so many people are turning to natural alternatives.

Inflammation – characterised by swelling, redness, pain and heat – underlies many diseases, probably a lot more than most of us realise. These include all the 'itis' conditions: arthritis, dermatitis, colitis, nephritis and hepatitis. Also included are asthma and others not usually associated with inflammation, such as Alzheimer's and Parkinson's (in which parts of the brain become inflamed), and atherosclerosis (in which the arteries become inflamed).

Pain and inflammation can be caused by an imbalance in a number of body processes, such as impaired liver detoxification, disturbed blood sugar control, allergies, excess oxidants, insufficient antioxidants and a lack of essential fats. Each of these can tip the body into a state of alarm. We'll be looking into each of these key factors, because simple diet and lifestyle changes can strengthen your body's resilience so that it won't be tipped into a state of inflammation.

YOUR PAIN LEVEL

Before we look at what happens in your body when pain occurs, and the mechanism behind painkilling drugs and natural painkilling nutrients and herbs, let's gauge your pain level.

Unlike a disease such as diabetes, which can be measured in the blood, there is no easy indicator in the blood for arthritis. The main indicator of pain and inflammation is simply how you feel. For this reason, health professionals use questionnaires to discover how effective a treatment is. There are several standard questionnaires, including the WOMAC (Western Ontario and McMaster Universities Osteoarthritis Index) check for hip and knee pain, and the Oswestry test for back and leg pain. Check yourself out on the questionnaire below.

Questionnaire: how's your pain?

Tick the box for yes or no, or add the score to the yes box where applicable.

		Yes	No
1	Do you have aching or painful joints?	☐	☐
2	Do you suffer from arthritis?	☐	☐
3	Do you have painful or aching muscles?	☐	☐
4	Do you suffer from muscle stiffness that limits your movement?	☐	☐
5	Do you wake up with physical pain?	☐	☐

6 Do you suffer from headaches? If so, how often? On average once a week (score 1), twice a week (score 2) or more (score 3)?   ☐ ☐

7 Does your level of pain make you feel tired?   ☐ ☐

8 Does pain make you feel weak?   ☐ ☐

9 Does it limit your ability to move around?   ☐ ☐

10 Does it limit your ability to sit for more than 30 minutes?   ☐ ☐

11 How intense is your pain, without medication? Mild (score 1); discomforting (score 2); distressing (score 3); horrible (score 4); excruciating (score 5)   ☐ ☐

Score 1 for each 'yes' answer, then add up your score.

Total score: ☐

Score
If your total score is:

Below 5 Your level of pain might be reduced by following the advice in this chapter. If not, I recommend you seek advice from a nutritional therapist or nutritionally oriented doctor.

Between 5 and 10 You have a moderate level of pain and should definitely explore each of the options in this chapter as well as seeking advice from a nutritional therapist or nutritionally oriented doctor.

More than 10 You have a high level of pain and I advise you to consult a nutritional therapist or nutritionally oriented doctor. Although exploring the options in this chapter will give you a good background, you may well need additional help to put it all into practice.

WHAT CAUSES PAIN AND INFLAMMATION AND HOW ARE THEY TREATED?

The substances that cause inflammation and pain are called 'inflammatory mediators', which your body produces in response to some sort of 'insult'. There are many of these body chemicals, such as prostaglandins, interleukins, cytokines, leukotrienes, oxidants, nitric oxide, insulin, and immunoglobulins. These in turn promote the accumulation of the substances that cause swelling, redness and pain.

Pain-causing prostaglandins and leukotrienes are made from one of the omega-6 fats, arachidonic acid, which is very high in meat and dairy products. Too much of these foods in your diet can lead to over-production of these pain-causing body chemicals. So it's a good reason to go easy on these foods if you're in pain. Although some degree of inflammation can be an important protective mechanism, too many inflammatory mediators create pain. This is because inflammation is an 'alarm signal' to alert the body that something is wrong.

All over the body there are chemical accelerators and brakes. In the case of inflammation, there are three critical enzymes that turn harmless arachidonic acid into harmful inflammatory mediators. These enzymes are called COX-1, COX-2 and 5-LOX, as shown in Figure 4 overleaf. You could think of COX-1 as the 'good' COX, because it helps to protect the gut and the kidneys and promotes normal blood clotting; however, COX-2 is the 'bad' one because it increases pain and swelling, but also thins the blood. Blocking COX-1 alone reduces pain but damages the gut and thins the blood. Blocking COX-2 alone reduces pain but increases blood clotting (this is examined in detail on pages 32–34). Non-steroidal anti-inflammatory drugs (NSAIDs for short), such as aspirin or ibuprofen, target both of these enzymes, so they are good for stopping pain and inflammation. On the minus side, though, they are also likely to put you at risk of gastrointestinal bleeding when used regularly over the long term, and they also tax the liver.

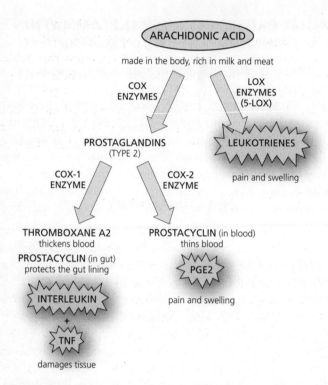

Figure 4 – How your body's chemistry makes pain

Because of the gastrointestinal problems mentioned above, the thinking was that the ideal NSAID would be one that blocked only COX-2 and left COX-1 alone. And the launch of drugs such as Vioxx in 1999 caused huge excitement because that's exactly what they did. But problems with these drugs began emerging a few years after they appeared on the scene. Blocking an element – such as an enzyme – that is part of a network as complex as the body almost never has just one effect, which is why drugs nearly always have damaging side effects.

In 2004, Merck voluntarily withdrew Vioxx from the market because of concerns about increased risk of heart attack and stroke associated with long-term, high-dosage use. The precise details of the case have been chewed over in the courts for years, but whatever the legal niceties it's clear that behind the scenes and in the medical literature, alarm bells had been ringing for years about the link with heart attacks. It's just that they had been deliberately ignored. You can read more about this shocking scandal in my book *Food is Better Medicine than Drugs*, with Jerome Burne (see Recommended Reading, page 343).

NEW DISCOVERY!

Scientists have focused on the COX-1 and COX-2 enzymes, but another pain-causing enzyme called 5-lipoxygenase (5-LOX) has been largely ignored. Scientists at the University of British Columbia found that combinations of COX and 5-LOX inhibitors were more effective than single inhibitors. Some nutrients – boswellic acid and curcumin, for example – have been found to inhibit this enzyme. Although 5-LOX is only just beginning to receive the attention it deserves among researchers, some pioneering work on the nature of this powerful enzyme suggests that levels tend to increase as we age.[7] What is even more exciting is that the effect of various nutrients working together is only just starting to become known. When you combine some nutrients in a certain way the pain-relieving effect is multiplied.

Using anti-inflammatory drugs in the short term can improve healing – as long as the problem that triggered the inflammation in the first place has gone. Eventually, if pain and inflammation persist over the long term, body tissues will begin to break down. In the case of arthritis, for example, the joint becomes increasingly hard and stiffened – calcified – until you can't use it at all.

If you have joint problems, you may have had your erythrocyte sedimentation rate (ESR) measured. A high ESR means

that your body is in a state of inflammation, as does a high level
of c-reactive protein (CRP).

How is inflammation usually treated?

The most common medical treatment for inflammation is
anti-inflammatory drugs. These drugs are effective symptom
suppressors, providing pain relief but doing nothing to address
the causes of the inflammation. According to Dr Jeffrey Bland,
a pioneer in new approaches to dealing with inflammation,
instead of thinking pain means drug, inflammation is the
body's way of saying something is wrong. Inflammation is a
systemic problem, not just a localised phenomenon, in which
the body's physiology is shifted into an 'alarm state'. It's as if
there is a series of underlying imbalances in the body's chemistry that build up and then burst forth, once the body can no
longer cope. The actual symptoms, or pain, are the wave breaking, but the wave is a long time coming.

THE UNDERLYING CAUSES OF INFLAMMATION

From this perspective, there are several factors that set the scene
for inflammation, and then there are those that trigger the
actual symptoms – which often get the blame. 'My arthritis
started when my marriage was breaking up', or 'Ever since I
had that bout of flu my joints started to ache.' These triggers
are important and may include a trauma, an allergy, an infection, a toxin or exposure to too many oxidants. However, a
healthy person can usually rise to such challenges. But if there
are underlying weaknesses, such as a genetic predisposition and
poor nutrition, the person may have no reserves in their 'health
bank' and so their body cannot respond to the slightest stress.

Inflammation can therefore be seen as the body's way of
showing that a person's total intake (including diet, drugs and

environmental chemicals) has exceeded their unique capacity to adapt, partly determined by their genes. The key factors that contribute to developing an inflammatory health problem are:

- Impaired liver detoxification capacity
- Disturbed blood sugar control
- Excess oxidants versus insufficient antioxidants
- Lack of essential fats
- Allergy

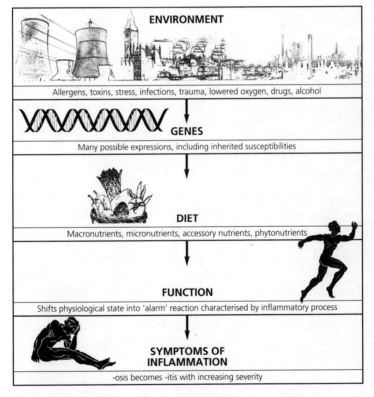

ENVIRONMENT

Allergens, toxins, stress, infections, trauma, lowered oxygen, drugs, alcohol

GENES

Many possible expressions, including inherited susceptibilities

DIET

Macronutrients, micronutrients, accessory nutrients, phytonutrients

FUNCTION

Shifts physiological state into 'alarm' reaction characterised by inflammatory process

SYMPTOMS OF INFLAMMATION

-osis becomes -itis with increasing severity

Figure 5 – The inflammatory process

HOW STRONG IS YOUR LIVER?

As a gastroenterologist from Harvard Medical School once said, 'A good stomach and a set of bowels are more important to human health and happiness than a large amount of brains.' The scene for inflammation may be set in the digestive tract, with faulty nutrition leading to dysbiosis (when healthy gut bacteria are disrupted), leading in turn to bacterial, fungal or parasitic infection, intestinal permeability (leaky gut) and allergy. Once the gut wall becomes 'leaky', more proteins get into the bloodstream, causing allergic reactions, and, along with other toxins, tax the liver's ability to detoxify. Once the liver's reserve is impaired, any dietary or environmental toxin can trigger inflammation.

The good news is that each of these factors can be tested and corrected – under the guidance of a nutritional therapist. Anyone with a long-term inflammatory problem such as arthritis is likely to benefit from seeing a nutritional therapist, having a liver detoxification test, and adjusting their diet as well as taking the appropriate supplements. This alone can make a real difference. This is discussed in more detail in Chapter 8.

ARE YOU INSULIN-DEPENDENT?

There is a strong link between many of the signs of inflammation and being resistant to insulin, the hormone produced by the pancreas that helps to control blood sugar levels. Most diabetics and overweight people are 'insulin-resistant' (meaning that their bodies don't react to insulin in the way that they should). Insulin is released into the bloodstream whenever you eat carbohydrates, especially sugar, or stimulants. The insulin then helps to transport the glucose from carbohydrates into body cells. If you are insulin-resistant (which is a hallmark of what's called metabolic syndrome or syndrome X) – the body has to produce even more insulin to get the same effect. As a consequence, glucose levels in the blood often go too high. Too much glucose or insulin in the blood is toxic and will trigger inflammatory reactions. In the cells, a disturbed glucose supply acts as a powerful oxidant, damaging cells, producing the symptom of fatigue and triggering inflammation, among other reactions. Then, as insulin starts to work, your blood sugar level can go too low, which triggers release of the stress hormone cortisol, again promoting inflammation. So it's vital to learn what to eat and drink to keep your blood sugar level even. This means:

- Eating more fibre in wholefoods, particularly soluble fibre (as found in oats, beans and vegetables).
- Eating foods that release their sugar content slowly (such as wholegrains, oats, lentils, beans, apples and raw or lightly cooked vegetables), called low–GL (glycemic load) foods. These are discussed in Chapter 7.
- Supplementing vitamin C (1,000mg), chromium (200mcg), and the essential fats, especially the fish oil EPA (1,200mg).

OXIDANTS VERSUS ANTIOXIDANTS

An inflammatory reaction is a state of alarm in the body. One of the body's primary defence weapons is oxidants, but these can also harm the body and initiate inflammation. It's a vicious circle. Oxidants are produced by the body in the mitochondria, the cells' energy factories, which turn glucose from food into energy. These oxidants, which are rather like toxic exhaust from an engine, must be rendered harmless by antioxidants such as vitamins A, C, E, selenium and zinc. Too many oxidants and not enough antioxidants can lead to cell damage.

The liver, too, produces oxidants if its detoxifying capacity has been exceeded. Another self-made oxidant is nitric oxide. Body levels of nitric oxide tend to be higher at times of inflammation and have been linked to arthritis. Although it has some important functions in the body, levels can become excessive and help to trigger inflammation if the immune system is already on red alert, perhaps due to frequent consumption of an allergen or through breathing in toxins. We also put oxidants into our bodies by eating fried food, smoking or breathing smoke-filled or polluted air. These can damage the gut or the lungs, leading to greater susceptibility to infection as well as inflammation.

That's why it's important to calm down the immune system by avoiding any allergens (more on this in Chapter 9), reduce sources of oxidants and increase your antioxidant nutrients (these nutrients are discussed fully in Chapter 10).

INFLAMMATORY FATS

The fats you eat can also promote or reduce inflammation. This is because special chemicals in the body, called prostaglandins, play a key role in the control of inflammation. These, in turn, are made from the fat you eat. The most beneficial kinds of fat are called essential fats and come in two families: omega-6 (high in sunflower, sesame and pumpkin seeds, borage oil and evening primrose oil) and omega-3 (high in oily fish and in flax seeds). EPA, an omega-3 fat found in oily fish, is especially anti-inflammatory. Supplementing evening primrose oil has proven as effective as anti-inflammatory drugs in the treatment of arthritis in some studies,[8] while numerous studies have reported less swelling, pain and tenderness after supplementing concentrated fish oils.[9] (Exactly what you need and why is covered in Chapter 6.)

ELIMINATING ALLERGIES

Most people with inflammatory diseases have allergies to certain foods or chemicals. These allergies may occur because of an inflamed gut wall, which allows large food proteins to pass through. Once these get into the body, they trigger an allergic response, which includes inflammation. The most common foods that produce allergies are dairy produce, wheat and other grains, as well as yeast, but you can become allergic to just about any food, especially if your gut wall has been damaged by taking NSAIDs.

One way to reduce the load on your digestive system is to find out what you're allergic to and avoid it for a period of time, to allow your digestive tract to heal. Many foods, if avoided for three months, can be reintroduced once the digestive tract is in good health, without triggering an allergic response. (The link between allergies and arthritis, and how to find out what you might be allergic to, is explained in Chapter 9.)

THE PAIN OF INFLAMMATION

These five factors together (digestion and detoxification problems, poor blood sugar control, too many oxidants versus a lack of antioxidants, lack of essential fats, and allergies) programme the body for inflammation. The substances that actually cause inflammation are called 'inflammatory mediators', as described earlier. Many of these substances also have beneficial roles to perform in the body, because inflammation is, after all, a necessary alarm signal. However, the presence of too many inflammatory mediators means you become primed for pain. Whereas drugs work by blocking these, the good news is that many natural remedies do too, without the side effects.

As explained, prostaglandins and leukotrienes are produced from arachidonic acid, which is found in meat and dairy products. One of the features of inflammation is increased oxygenation of arachidonic acid, which then leads to the production of prostaglandins and leukotrienes, which trigger pain and inflammation. NSAID drugs work by blocking the production of these inflammatory substances, but not without side effects.

Going natural

There are natural ways to reduce inflammation even more effectively than the ways mentioned above and without the side effects. These include taking herbs and food extracts such as curcumin from turmeric, hop extracts, the herb boswellia, something in olives called hydroxytyrosol, quercetin, which is found in red onions and apples among other foods (more on these in Chapter 5), and anti-inflammatory essential fats from seeds and fish. These will become the backbone of your natural anti-inflammatory strategy, allowing you to reduce your use of pain-killing drugs. In the next chapter I'll explain why it's a good idea to do this.

CHAPTER 4

....

WHY PAINKILLERS DON'T WORK LONG TERM

There's a good and a bad side to inflammation and to the drugs used to treat it. When it first appears, it's a sign that your body is responding to a problem and trying to deal with it. It's the way we fight off infections, for instance. But if an area is still inflamed after the problem has been dealt with, it can get in the way of healing. When this happens, using anti-inflammatory drugs in the short term can improve healing – as long as the problem that triggered the inflammation in the first place has gone. If it hasn't, then taking anti-inflammatory drugs for any length of time just allows you to ignore the underlying causes. In the case of arthritis, this could be a food allergy, a lack of omega-3 fats or a physical misalignment.

PAIN AND PAINKILLERS – DOUBLE-EDGED SWORDS

As I mentioned above, the most common medical treatment for inflammation is to take anti-inflammatory drugs. Although these are effective symptom suppressors, which provide pain relief, they do nothing to address the causes of the inflammation. They don't just mask the problem, however, they are also dangerous, as I'll explain later.

What are they called?

Anti-inflammatories are available in several forms, but by far the most commonly used are NSAIDs, which include aspirin, ibuprofen (common name, Nurofen), flurbiprofen (Froben), ketoprofen (Orudis, Oruvail), naproxen (Naprosyn), sulindac (Clinoril), indomethacin (Indocid), mefenamic acid (Ponstan), diclofenac (Voltarol), oxaprozin (Daypro), salsalate (Amigesic, Disalcid), etodolac (Ultradol), nabumetone (Relafen, Relifex) and piroxicam (Feldene). Celecoxib (Celebrex) also comes under the heading of NSAIDs and is in a class of medications known as selective COX-2 inhibitors. In more severe cases of rheumatoid arthritis, glucocorticoids or so-called 'disease-modifying anti-rheumatic drugs' (DMARDs) may be prescribed. DMARDs either affect the immune response (for example, gold, penicillamine, methotrexate and chloroquine) or suppress the disease process (for example, sulphasalazine). Also used for rheumatoid arthritis and other autoimmune conditions are anti-tumour necrosis factor (TNF) agents, including infliximab and etanercept. Because of their potential toxicity, treatment with these drugs is prescribed only by specialist rheumatologists, and they are therefore not covered in detail in this book.

What do they do?

Prescriptions for NSAIDs cost the UK's National Health Service about £250 million a year. They work by blocking the production of the body's inflammatory mediators, but, although they are mostly very effective for pain relief, they are not without side effects, especially in the gut (see the chart opposite).

The risks

NSAIDs are responsible for many toxic reactions and often cause undesirable side effects, including headaches, dizziness

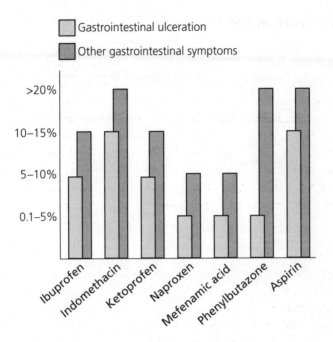

Figure 6 – NSAID side effects

and digestive complaints such as nausea, vomiting, diarrhoea and intestinal bleeding. They can also cause kidney damage.[10] Their use should therefore be recommended only for short periods of time, if at all.[11] NSAIDs have also been associated with increased gut permeability and ulcers in the small intestine, which can have serious complications.[12] It has been suggested that a large proportion of hitherto unexplained ulcers in the small intestine could be due to these drugs.[13]

At least nine NSAID drugs have been withdrawn from use, including Opren. Approximately one-quarter of all adverse drug reactions reported are for this group of drugs. In the US,

NSAIDs are an $8.5 billion dollar industry: $6.5 billion for the drugs and $2 billion for treating the side effects.[14]

It may seem extraordinary, but this class of drug is responsible for more deaths than any other. Of the 10,000 or more deaths in the UK every year from prescribed drugs, anti-inflammatory drugs account for about a quarter. In the US, the figure is 16,500 deaths a year – more than from asthma, cervical cancer or malignant melanoma.[15]

The other, more heavyweight drugs are the corticosteroids such as prednisone. They are based on the steroid cortisone (hence the phrase 'non-steroidal' to distinguish the aspirin-type drugs) and can be very dangerous over the long term. This is because they suppress the production of cortisol, the body's natural anti-inflammatory hormone, which is reserved for emergencies and acts as an immediate painkiller following serious accidents. More about these later.

The long-term use of painkillers is also associated with 'chronic daily headache'. Painkillers should never be taken more than one day in four, or seven days a month. When used long term, NSAIDs such as aspirin and ibruprofen can cause gastrointestinal bleeding and can put a strain on the liver. Recent studies have also shown that new anti-inflammatory drugs, which inhibit important enzymes, can double or in some cases quadruple a person's chance of a heart attack.[16] Despite this danger the average person takes in excess of 300 doses of these painkillers a year! That's six a week.

WHY SOME NSAIDS CAUSE HEART PROBLEMS

As we saw in the previous chapter (page 19), COX-1 can be thought of as the 'good' COX, because it helps to protect the gut and the kidneys and promotes normal blood clotting, whereas COX-2 is the 'bad' one because it leads to the painful prostaglandins. One of the first NSAIDs was aspirin, which targets both of these enzymes. Thus it's good for stopping pain and inflammation, but it's also likely to put patients at risk by causing gastrointestinal bleeding when used over the long term, and it also taxes the liver. Ibuprofen also targets both enzymes.

As illustrated in Figure 4 in the previous chapter, the COX-1 pathway, besides making mucus to protect the guts (prostacyclin), also makes a fat-like substance called thromboxane A2. This promotes the narrowing of blood vessels and makes blood cells called platelets more 'sticky'. The COX-2 pathway, on the other hand, makes what might be thought of as the antidote – a substance called prostacyclin, which helps prevent platelets from clumping together and helps to dilate the blood vessels.

In a healthy system, the action of these two would be balanced. But as illustrated in Figure 7, inhibiting COX-1 and/or COX-2 reduces pain but also leads to side effects. By powerfully inhibiting the COX-2 pathway (and so blocking prostacyclin in the blood, leading to increased blood clotting), the new generation of so-called 'coxib' drugs (like Vioxx, see page 20) created a fresh problem, doubling, or in some cases quadrupling, a person's risk of a heart attack.[17] This effect of coxibs also caused another problem, increasing the level of damage to brain cells in the event of a stroke.[18]

These 'new-generation', 'safer' painkillers were principally designed for patients who were at increased risk of gastrointestinal damage from NSAIDs. However, according to a study by researchers at the University of Chicago, '63% of the growth in COX-2 use occurred in patients with minimal risk of suffering gastrointestinal bleeding with NSAIDs.'[19]

Most people are not even aware of these awful risks.

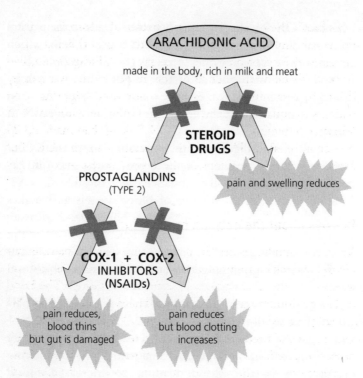

Figure 7 – How COX-1 and COX-2 painkillers induce side effects

Case Study: Robert

Robert is a case in point. 'I've had two heart attacks in the last four months,' says 57-year-old Robert. He had been taking Vioxx for four years, during which time his blood pressure rose and he began to have chest pains. 'I have no history of heart problems in my family,' he says. 'No one warned me about any dangers of heart attacks. I'm not taking anything for my arthritis now and getting out of bed in the morning can be murder.'

Because these drugs were no better at controlling pain, there was probably no benefit to switching to them at all. In fact, the decision to prescribe them, say the Chicago team, 'had nothing to do with science or the evidence but was simply driven by heavy marketing and the tendency of physicians and patients to equate newer with better'. Until the withdrawal of Vioxx in September 2004, the COX-2 drugs had made up 25 per cent of all NSAID drugs prescribed in the UK, but accounted for 50 per cent of the costs.[20] These were highly profitable drugs.

Worries about the new kid on the block

What is astounding is that the drug Arcoxia (generic name etoricoxib), Merck's proposed replacement for Vioxx, is not yet approved in the US but has been approved in Europe. The Food and Drug Administration (FDA) issued Merck a 'non-approvable letter' for Arcoxia in April 2007, stating that Merck needs to provide more test results showing that Arcoxia's benefits outweigh its risks before it has another chance of getting approved. However, Arcoxia is available in over 60 other countries, including the UK. (The list of potential side effects makes for extremely worrying reading.) So, people in the US have no choice; they can't have it. But Europeans can have it with a health warning!

However, it isn't just coxib drugs you need be concerned about. As a study published in 2005 shows, other NSAIDs, including ibuprofen, can also raise the risk of heart attacks, although not by as much as Vioxx.[21] A study in Spain in 2006 showed that NSAIDs can increase the risk of heart failure by 30 per cent.[22]

BACK TO ASPIRIN?

Given the dangers of COX-2 inhibitor painkillers, should we be switching back to aspirin, which also blocks COX-1?

Unfortunately, it looks like a case of out of the frying pan into the fire. Out of every 1,000 people aged 55 to 59 who take a low-dose daily aspirin to prevent heart attack, about two will be prevented from getting a heart attack. But that comes at a high price.

Aspirin side effects

The amount of aspirin often needed to make a difference to inflammation is relatively high (2–4g a day), so toxic side effects do occur. The early warning signs of toxicity include tinnitus and gastric irritation. Aspirin is an unnatural substance for the human body, which reacts to it as an irritant.

The effect of preventing heart attacks is about evenly weighted with the risk of having serious gastrointestinal problems: two in 1,000 will suffer a major gastrointestinal bleed by age 60.[23] In 1980, the sixth World Nutrition Congress reported that even a single aspirin can cause intestinal bleeding for one week in some people. Just imagine what high doses on a daily basis over many years are likely to do.

Many other NSAIDs also cause gastrointestinal symptoms, including ulcers, which kill several thousand people in the UK every year.[24] (In the UK, there are 25 million annual NSAID prescriptions, 12,000 hospital admissions and 2,600 related deaths.) One small study published in 2005, using new scanning technology, has recently found that NSAIDs may damage more than the stomach. Seventy per cent of patients who had been taking NSAIDs for just three months had visible damage to their small intestine.[25]

One other side effect of aspirin and some other NSAIDs that is rarely mentioned is that they can actually make the damage caused by arthritis worse. They stop the production of the collagen and other materials in the matrix that, with minerals and water, make up the substance of bone; and in the process they speed up the destruction of cartilage in joints.[26]

They can also worsen the key problem arthritis sufferers are wrestling with in another way: aspirin lowers blood levels of vitamin C, which is vital for the formation of collagen.

So, in the short term, the use of aspirin may relieve symptoms, but in the long term it is more likely to cause further problems. Please note, however, that NSAIDs should be reduced slowly, as an abrupt end to medication often makes symptoms flare up.

PARACETAMOL AND THE LIVER

Paracetamol, called acetaminophen in the US, works in a different way from NSAIDs. Although it can reduce pain, it lacks anti-inflammatory activity. There is little evidence that it suppresses the COX enzyme, or that its analgesic effect comes from reducing inflammation and swelling. Instead, as a study from 2000 shows, it seems to mainly reduce pain by boosting chemicals called opioids in the brain, making you less sensitive to the pain. [27]

An Australian study from 2004 showed that 66 per cent of patients found that paracetamol was better than ibuprofen, aspirin or the newer and much more expensive COX-2 inhibitors.[28] However, most studies on arthritic patients have shown the opposite: that it is less effective than other NSAIDs.[29]

Paracetamol side effects

The problem with paracetamol is that it is notoriously toxic to the liver, an effect which lands thousands of people in the UK in hospital each year, kills several hundred and is a major cause of the need for liver transplants.[30] According to Professor Sir David Carter, director of the Liver Transplant Centre at Edinburgh Royal Infirmary, one in ten liver transplants is due to damage caused by paracetamol overdose.[31]

THE CORTISONE DILEMMA

All of this brings us back to the original 'miracle' painkiller: cortisone and the subsequent steroid-based drugs such as prednisone, prednisolone and betamethasone. Cortisone is a derivative of a hormone produced naturally by the body in the adrenal cortex, which sits on top of each kidney.

Steroid-based drugs were the most commonly prescribed treatment for arthritic conditions back in the 1980s. Since the discovery of cortisone more than 40 years ago, 101 uses have been found for it, including the relief of pain and the treatment of arthritis.

Back in 1948 Philip S. Hench, who later won a Nobel Prize, reported miraculous results using cortisone on arthritis suffers disabled by the condition. But the hope that it was a cure for arthritis didn't last long. In one early case, a 10-year-old girl – who had made an amazing recovery from severe arthritis when given cortisone – quickly developed diabetes. When the cortisone was stopped, the diabetes melted away – and the arthritis returned with a vengeance. Even so, 29 million prescriptions for cortisone are written for arthritis each year in the US.

It's still not completely understood exactly how cortisone works. It's known that it brings down inflammation by stopping production of the inflammatory compound histamine. It also suppresses the immune system, which could be good if your immune system is destroying healthy cells, as in an autoimmune disease like rheumatoid arthritis. And, in addition, it blocks COX-2, which seems to be the main way it relieves pain.

Cortisone side effects

The trouble is that once you start taking cortisone, the adrenal glands stop producing it. Given in small amounts, cortisone seems manageable; but in large amounts, particularly over long periods of time, it causes disastrous and even deadly side effects.

The sad truth is that, like aspirin, cortisone does not cure anything. 'It merely suppresses the symptoms of the disease,' says Dr Barnett Zumoff of Beth Israel Medical Center in New York City, and formerly of the Steroid Research Laboratory at New York's Montefiore Hospital.[32] Withdrawal from high doses of cortisone must be very gradual to allow the adrenal glands to start producing their own cortisone again. Even so, a full recovery is often not possible, leaving previous cortisone users unable to produce enough to respond to stressful situations such as an accident or operation. Severe adrenal insufficiency can be fatal. Congestive heart failure can also result from long-term use.

Some of the other consequences of taking this drug over a long period of time may not be fatal, but they can certainly be extremely unpleasant. They include obesity, a rounded 'moon' face, a higher susceptibility to infection, slow wound healing and muscle wasting. 'Using it,' says Dr Zumoff, 'is like trying to repair a computer with a monkey wrench.' Although cortisone has undoubtedly saved many lives, it is unlikely to cure arthritis if taken over months or years, and may even speed up the disease because it can weaken cartilage and remove minerals from bone.[33]

PAINKILLERS – DO THE BENEFITS OUTWEIGH THE RISKS?

From any rational perspective, it's clear that none of the anti-inflammatories I've described are safe for handling joint pain in the long term. But does their effectiveness outweigh the risks?

A review of 23 trials, including one involving 10,845 patients with arthritic knee pain, published in a 2004 issue of the *British Medical Journal* concludes: 'NSAIDs can reduce short term pain in osteoarthritis of the knee slightly better than placebo, but the current analysis does not support long term use of NSAIDs for this condition. As serious adverse effects are associated with oral NSAIDs, only limited use can be recommended.'[34] In a long-term trial, NSAIDs taken over one to four years were no better than a placebo.

So, taking painkillers looks a risky business, long term. If you over-block COX-1 you get intestinal bleeding and kidney problems; if you over-block COX-2 you increase your risk of blood clots and having a heart attack. Among the most dangerous are aspirin, diclofenac, ibuprofen, ketoprofen and naproxen, and the coxib drug celecoxib. Paracetamol (or acetaminophen) overdose accounts for over half of the cases of liver failure and death. In some combinations (such as taking aspirin with ibuprofen), these drugs can become even more dangerous.[35] Using them long term when there are other, safer, nutrition-based options seems perverse.

NATURE DOES IT BETTER THAN DRUGS

As I'll show you in the following chapter, there are natural ways to reduce inflammation that are as effective as drugs (if not more so), with fewer side effects. However, the real answer to inflammation involves tackling its underlying causes, rather than just treating the symptoms. It is also important to supplement nutrients that support the rebuilding of damaged joints (see Chapter 16). This new approach to conquering inflammation is complex, like the problem itself, and is best achieved by working with a nutritional therapist who can run the necessary tests and advise you on diet and supplements for each stage of reprogramming the body. This approach is based on an understanding that inflammation and pain is the body's way of saying 'Help!' and that current diet and lifestyle factors have exceeded the body's capacity to adapt. Such a strategy can normally be completed in three to six months, leading to a significant reduction in pain.

Case Study: Ed

Ed is a case in point. He first started getting joint pain in his mid-thirties. He had kept himself fit by playing tennis daily and running, often on hard pavements, before the days of air-filled trainers. After an accident in which he tore a ligament, he needed surgery, which revealed that the cartilage in his knee was severely damaged. The damaged cartilage was surgically removed. A few years later the same thing happened to his other knee. And, a few years on, he needed a second operation on the first knee! Now, in his mid-forties, and three surgeries later he was suffering from severe arthritis, with ever-increasing pain. When the body goes into a state of inflammation, trying to immobilise a damaged knee, it actually causes more and more damage to the cartilage, especially if the joint in question is a weight-bearing joint, such as the knees, hips or lower back.

Ed's job as a vice-president at Merrill Lynch kept him active and took him travelling all over the world. He also liked to keep fit playing golf. He liked walking and adventurous holidays but, increasingly, the pain in his knees was slowing him down and grounding him. He tried wearing a brace, applying heat treatments and taking numerous anti-inflammatory drugs, from Advil to Vioxx, but his knees just got worse and worse until he could no longer play a round of golf without being in excruciating pain afterwards and having to lie down for an hour or so, waiting for the pain to ease. He had the best that medicine could offer, but it wasn't making any difference. In fact, he was getting worse. He couldn't travel so much, couldn't play tennis any more and could barely play golf even with a golf cart. I met him five years ago, at the age of 57. He said he'd do anything to get some relief. I told him to read the original edition of this book from cover to cover and to do everything it says, and I gave him a list of supplements to take. There was little improvement in the first two months, but by the third month his knees were feeling a whole lot better. By six months he was virtually pain-free.

> 'I used to have constant pain in my knees and joints, could not play golf or walk more than 10 minutes without resting my legs. Since following your advice my discomfort has decreased 95–100 per cent. It is a different life when you can travel and play golf every day. I never would have believed my pain could be reduced by such a large degree, and not return, no matter how much activity in a day or week.'

Now, five years on, Ed remains 95 per cent pain-free and has had no return or worsening of his symptoms – and he needs no medication. Recently he told me that he can play two rounds of golf a day without experiencing any pain and plays a round most days.

> 'At the age of 62 I'm hitting the golfball as far and as good as I ever have in my life. I have great flexibility and show no signs of ageing.'

Ed is living proof that the body can heal itself if you give it the right nutrients, whatever your age. In the next part I'll explain the key components to a natural anti-inflammatory strategy.

PART 2

REDUCING INFLAMMATION AND PAIN

CHAPTER 5

NATURAL PAINKILLERS

Antioxidants, herbs and spices are important ingredients in a healthy diet. What's less well known is that, judiciously chosen, they're also effective at treating joint pain. This may sound beyond the pale. After all, if they were, the experts would be recommending them – right? Unfortunately, there are strong commercial reasons why scepticism about this approach remains widespread. And you have to remember that scepticism is quite different from a lack of evidence. Herbs and vitamins, unlike drugs, can't be patented and are therefore vastly under-researched and under-marketed. What's more, the law specifically prohibits herbal and supplement companies from describing any of the benefits of the supplements they sell in their catalogues or websites. Different combinations of these herbs and nutrients are likely to be particularly powerful anti-inflammatories and painkillers.

Of the natural anti-inflammatory agents that have proven to be effective, with minimal, if any, side effects, the most interesting are:

- Curcumin (found in turmeric)
- Boswellic acid (found in Indian frankincense)
- Ashwagandha
- Flavonoids, especially quercetin (found in tea, red onions, apples and some citrus fruits)

- Ginger
- Bromelain (found in pineapples)
- Hop extracts
- Hydroxytyrosol, found in olives

CURCUMIN

The bright yellow pigment of the spice turmeric contains the active compound curcumin, which has a variety of powerful anti-inflammatory actions. Studies show it works as well as anti-inflammatory drugs, but without the side effects.[1] Like NSAIDs, it blocks the formation of the pro-inflammatory prostaglandins (type 2), as well as leukotrienes (see Figure 8, on page 48).[2] In fact, it turns out to be what everyone hoped drugs like Vioxx would be: a mild 5-LOX and COX-2 inhibitor that not does not affect COX-1. What's more, it has been used for its medicinal properties in Ayurveda (Indian traditional medicine) for hundreds of years. There is no evidence of any downsides, even in high doses of 8g a day. It also mops up nitric oxide (another inflammatory mediator) and is a powerful antioxidant. In addition, it has been shown to promote detoxification.

Interestingly, the most recent review of turmeric in the *Journal of Clinical Immunology* states that curcumin at low doses can also enhance antibody responses.[3] This suggests that curcumin's reported beneficial effects in arthritis, allergies, asthma, atherosclerosis, heart disease, Alzheimer's and cancer might be due in part to its ability to modulate the immune system. I highly recommend it for both osteoarthritis and rheumatoid arthritis.

Astonishingly, a US company tried to get a patent on turmeric in 1995, claiming it was a 'new' discovery for the treatment of inflammation. But the Indian government successfully challenged this on the grounds that the spice had been used for precisely that purpose in India for generations.

How to use it

Use turmeric in cooking for its great flavour in curries and stir-fries, or add a teaspoon when cooking rice. The only downside is that it can stain, so take care when using in cooking. A heaped teaspoon a day will do the trick, or you can buy supplements, in which case you'll need about 300–500mg, one to three times a day.

BOSWELLIA

Frankincense may be the ultimate gift for an arthritic friend, because *Boswellia serrata*, also known as Indian frankincense, is a very powerful natural anti-inflammatory agent, without the side effects of current drugs.[4] Boswellic acids contained in this herb achieve comparative anti-inflammatory effects without the associated gut problems of anti-inflammatory and painkilling drugs such as aspirin. In one study, where patients initially received boswellic acid and then later a placebo, arthritic symptoms were significantly reduced while taking the boswellia, but returned when the treatment was switched over to the placebo.[5]

Boswellic acid appears to reduce joint swelling, restores and improves blood supply to inflamed joints, provides pain relief and increased mobility, and improves morning stiffness. Not only does it perform all these actions through its anti-inflammatory effect, but it also seems to protect the actual substance of joints by preventing or slowing down the breakdown of cartilage. When components of soft tissue are broken down or 'chipped away', inflammation is initiated, followed by destruction of the joint. Boswellia appears to prevent or slow the breakdown of the components of cartilage, so it may play an important part in a cartilage-rebuilding regime, discussed more fully in Chapter 16. Trials with arthritic patients have shown significant relief after four weeks supplementing 600mg of boswellic acid.[6] It works in a different way from turmeric and other COX-2 inhibitors, which is why I like to use a combination of boswellia and a potent COX-2 inhibitor such as curcumin, or the hop extract IsoOxygene.

How to use it

Preparations of boswellia are available in tablet and cream form. With supplements, the ideal dose is 200–400mg, once or twice a day. Creams are especially useful in the treatment of localised inflammation (see Anti-inflammatory Gels and Creams, page 55).

ASHWAGANDHA

The herb ashwagandha (*Withania somnifera*) is a promising natural remedy that has been also used for hundreds of years as part of Ayurvedic medicine. The active ingredients of this powerful, natural anti-inflammatory herb are called withanolides. These inhibit COX-2 and also appear to have anti-cancer properties.[7] In one study, 42 patients with osteoarthritis were found to have a significant reduction in pain and disability after taking a formula containing ashwagandha, boswellia, turmeric and zinc for three months.[8]

How to use it

The therapeutic dose depends on the concentration of with-anolides. Try 300–500mg twice a day of the ashwagandha root, providing 1.5 per cent withanolides.

QUERCETIN

There is more truth to the expression 'an apple a day keeps the doctor away' than you might think! Apples are a good source of quercetin, which is a naturally occurring bioflavonoid increasingly used in the treatment of inflammatory diseases.

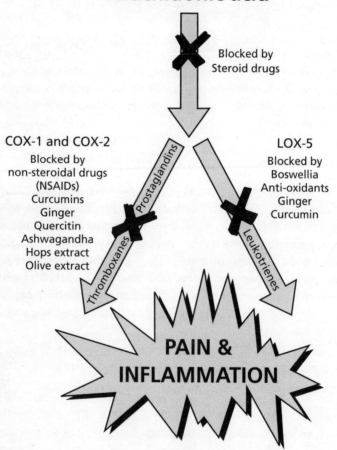

Figure 8 – How NSAIDs, boswellia and curcumins
reduce inflammation

(Bioflavonoids, which are the compounds that give fruits and vegetables their colour, are frequently found in nature alongside vitamin C; that is, fruits and vegetables that contain flavonoids are generally also rich in vitamin C.) Many plant foods contain flavonoid compounds, which are known to inhibit inflammation.[9] These are found in fruits and vegetables, especially in red/blue foods such as berries and beetroot, as well as red onions. One red onion, or a cup of berries, or three servings of greens provides about 10mg of quercetin. Other good sources of quercetin include red wine, tea, grapefruit, broccoli, squash, red grapes, cranberries and citrus fruits. This is one reason why vegetarian diets have proven highly effective in reducing pain and inflammation.

Quercetin is a potent anti-inflammatory and one of the most abundant antioxidants.[10] It works with vitamin C and E to protect against free radical damage and also helps stabilise cells and reduce the breakdown of collagen (the material needed by the body to maintain healthy joint tissue) – all of which are important in the management of arthritis. Although I know of no trials so far that have been conducted on arthritis, all the evidence on quercetin's effects on the body's biochemistry are encouraging. It has been shown to inhibit the production of the pro-inflammatory prostaglandins (type 2)[11] and also inhibits the release of histamine, which is involved in inflammatory reactions.

How to use it

Quercetin is available in health-food stores as a stand-alone supplement as well as in some combination formulas. Take 300–600mg per day, between meals.

GINGER

The spice ginger is another effective anti-inflammatory favoured by Ayurvedic medicine for thousands of years. The learned doctors of this ancient and respected tradition knew that ginger was highly beneficial for reducing inflammation and rheumatism, but they probably didn't know why. Now 20th-century technology has demonstrated that ginger inhibits the synthesis of pro-inflammatory prostaglandins and thromboxanes, another type of inflammatory mediator.[12] It also has strong antioxidant properties, helping to mop up free radicals or prevent them from being generated (as discussed in Chapter 10), and is often used for travel and morning sickness due to its anti-emetic properties.[13]

Supplementing ginger in one study reduced the pain and swelling of three-quarters of the participants with osteoarthritis, while all patients with muscular discomfort experienced relief from pain.[14] (There was a good safety profile, with mostly mild gastro-intestinal adverse events in the ginger extract group.)

How to use it

Taking a supplement of 500–2,000mg of ginger a day is ideal. Otherwise, incorporate a 1cm (½in) slice of fresh ginger into your daily diet.

BROMELAIN

A collection of enzymes, bromelain is found in pineapples. Since it was first used in 1957, it has been shown to have a wide variety of medicinal properties – including the reduction of inflammation in rheumatoid arthritis.

There are several mechanisms by which bromelain is believed to help. Firstly, it inhibits pro-inflammatory compounds and blocks the production of kinins: compounds that increase swelling and cause pain. Secondly, it helps reduce swelling by breaking down fibrin: a mesh that forms around an inflamed area, blocking off the blood supply and impairing tissue drainage.

How to use it

Bromelain can be taken in supplement form: 200–400mg a day in between meals (that is, mid-morning and mid-afternoon).

HOPS EXTRACT

Those who think of hops only as an ingredient in beer might be surprised to know it provides one of the most effective natural painkillers of all. An extract from hops, called IsoOxygene, is one of the most potent natural COX-2 inhibitors and therefore one of the most effective natural painkillers. It works just as well as painkilling drugs, as has been shown in a recent study comparing the effects of IsoOxygene to ibuprofen. Two tablets of ibuprofen inhibited COX-2 by 62 per cent, whereas IsoOxygene achieved a 56 per cent inhibition.[15] Not only is it almost as effective as ibuprofen but it also doesn't have the gut-related side effects of anti-inflammatory drugs. This is because ibuprofen also inhibits COX-1 (the so-called 'good' COX, as it produces prostacyclin, which protects the gut lining), whereas IsoOxygene does not. Comparatively, IsoOxygene had almost a sixth of the inhibitory effect on COX-1.

How to use it

You need between 400mg and 800mg a day of hops extract.

MARVEL OF THE MED: OLIVE EXTRACT

Olives contain two natural painkillers. The first is called hydroxytyrosol, which has very powerful antioxidant and anti-inflammatory effects. The active ingredients in this extract are called polyphenols: plant chemicals that give some fruit and vegetables their colour. Red grapes and red onions (both of which also contain the natural anti-inflammatory quercetin) contain polyphenols, as does green tea. But with an antioxidant content over ten times greater than that of vitamin C, none of these are as powerful as hydroxytyrosol.

The polyphenol in hydroxytyrosol isn't the end of the story. Olives and their oil contain another compound called oleocanthal, which is chemically related to ibuprofen, although it has none of the negative side effects. This is the ingredient that gives olive oil a throaty bite, like a slight sting at the back of the mouth, just as ibuprofen does. In 2005, researchers at the Monell Chemical Senses Center and University of the Sciences in the US found that oleocanthal was a potent anti-inflammatory painkiller[16] that partially inhibits the activity of the COX-1 and COX-2 enzymes.

Like boswellia and turmeric, olive extract decreases levels of pro-inflammatory substances. Studies on olive pulp extract have shown that it reduces levels of two inflammatory messengers called TNF-alpha and interleukin-8. In fact one study with mice found that the extract reduced TNF-alpha levels by 95 per cent.[17] However, a combination of olive pulp extract, hop extracts, other herbs such as turmeric or boswellia, and omega-3 fish oils (as explained in Chapter 6) and antioxidants, is the best way forward because it will tackle pain and inflammation on several fronts at once.

How to use it

Although eating olives will give you a small amount of the extract, taking a supplement containing concentrated olive extract is a guaranteed way of getting enough. Aim for 400mg a day of olive extract. I also recommend increasing your intake of all antioxidants by taking two antioxidant complex supplements daily, plus 2g of vitamin C (to be discussed further in Chapter 10).

PHENYLALANINE

Although it is not an anti-inflammatory as such, the amino acid phenylalanine is an effective painkiller in much the same way that codeine or paracetamol affect painkilling messages in the brain.

The body also has the ability to produce immensely powerful pain inhibitors, known as opioid peptides, such as enkephalins. These are morphine-like natural painkillers in our bodies, like endorphins, which produce the so-called 'runners high'. These substances are 10 to 1,000 times more potent than morphine but, unfortunately, their action is short lived. Dl-phenylalanine has been shown to extend their life span by inhibiting the enzymes that break them down. Phenylalanine comes in two forms: d-phenylalanine (DPA), or dl-phenylalanine (DLPA). Being natural constituents of food, DPA and DLPA can be bought as supplements in health-food stores. DPA and DLPA have proved effective in relieving chronic pain, even when standard medication has given limited or no relief.

Unlike painkilling drugs, the benefit of DLPA and DPA is gradual and builds up over weeks. In one study, 43 patients, mainly with osteoarthritis, were given 250mg of DPA three to four times daily for four to five weeks. Significant pain reduction was reported among osteoarthritis sufferers, especially during the last two weeks.[18] In another study, in which 21 chronic pain sufferers were given either placebo pills or DPA, seven patients on DPA experienced 50 per cent pain relief, which was not maintained when they were switched on to a placebo. The remaining 13 patients had no significant relief of pain from DPA.[19] These studies followed up an earlier study, which had shown between good and total relief of pain in a group of ten patients, including those with osteoarthritis, rheumatoid arthritis and low back pain after only three days on DPA.[20]

However, not all studies have shown benefit from the use of DPA or DLPA.[21] Results suggest that the effects are cumulative and may appear only after two weeks of supplementation in some cases. Some people seem to obtain good pain relief from DPA or DLPA, whereas others do not. One 47-year-old woman, who had suffered with rheumatoid arthritis for 18 years – with severe swelling of the hands to the point where you couldn't see her knuckles – tried DLPA. Within seven days the pain and swelling reduced so dramatically that her knuckles were visible and her joints became flexible.[22]

How to use it

The recommended dose is 250mg of DPA (or 750mg of DLPA) three times a day for three weeks. If this dose is ineffective, you may wish to try a higher dose, but this should not be done without the supervision of your doctor or a qualified nutritional therapist, as high doses of amino acids can also have side effects. Side effects associated with excessive DPA or DLPA include increased anxiety, high blood pressure and headaches. Because amino acids in protein within food compete with each other for absorption into the body, DPA and DLPA are best taken at least 15–30 minutes before a meal on an empty stomach or with juice.

USING FORMULAS

The easiest way to supplement all these natural antiinflammatory agents is in various combined herbal formulas. Since their effect is probably synergistic, this may prove more effective than taking just one ingredient alone. Some examples of good formulas are given in Resources (see page 348). The two most important natural anti-inflammatory agents are curcumin and boswellia. These can also be found in creams that can be applied locally, reducing pain and swelling in specific joints.

ANTI-INFLAMMATORY GELS AND CREAMS

There are a number of anti-inflammatory creams and gels available that can be applied locally, reducing pain and swelling in specific joints, such as the hands and knees.

Arnica One of the most popular gels is arnica (*Arnica montana*), a medicinal herb that has been used for centuries to relieve pain and inflammation. Swiss researchers divided 204 patients with osteoarthritis of the hands into two groups and instructed them to rub either arnica gel or ibuprofen gel into their affected joints three times a day. The arnica gel was found to be as effective as the ibuprofen gel; three weeks later there were similar improvements in both groups in terms of pain, grip strength and other measures of hand function.[23] *Arnica montana* gel was also found to be safe, well tolerated, and effective for osteoarthritis of the knee when applied twice daily for six weeks.[24]

Celadrin (see page 67) is another anti-inflammatory that is available as a cream and has been found to be very effective for osteoarthritis of the knee when applied twice daily, in the morning and evening. It has been shown to improve the range of motion as well as the ability to walk up and down stairs and to rise from a sitting position.[25] By reducing pain, it also improved knee-osteoarthritis patients' ability to stand.[26] And it works very quickly: after only one week of twice-daily treatment with Celadrin cream, patients with arthritis and severe pain in the knee, elbow or wrist had reduced pain and improved mobility in all three joints![27]

Capsaicin (pronounced 'cap-*say*-sin') is the active ingredient in chilli peppers. Capsaicin cream, also called capsicum cream, is used for the temporary relief of painful muscles and joints associated with arthritis as well as simple backache, strains and sprains. Capsaicin reduces the amount of a natural chemical known as substance P (a neurochemical that transmits pain), which is present in painful joints. Substance P is believed to be involved in two processes central to arthritis: the release of enzymes that produce inflammation, and the transmission of pain impulses from the joints to the central nervous system. By blocking the production and release of substance P, capsaicin can reduce the pain associated with arthritis as well as dampen the transmission of pain messages to the brain. Capsaicin cream produces a temporary reduction in pain, so it must be used regularly to provide prolonged pain relief.

Researchers with Case Western Reserve University found that capsaicin cream worked better than a placebo in 70 osteoarthritis patients and 31 with rheumatoid arthritis. After four weeks of applying capsaicin cream (0.025 per cent) or placebo to painful knees, the capsaicin patients had significantly more pain relief: rheumatoid arthritis patients had 57 per cent pain reduction and osteoarthritis patients had 33 per cent pain reduction.[28]

Capsaicin cream (0.075 per cent) was also effective for the treatment of painful hand joints when applied four times daily for four weeks. This double blind, placebo-controlled, randomized trial (RCT) involved 21 patients with rheumatoid arthritis or osteoarthritis. However, capsaicin reduced tenderness and pain associated with osteoarthritis, but not rheumatoid arthritis compared with the placebo. A local burning sensation was the only adverse effect noted.[29]

How much to use A typical dosage is 0.025 per cent capsaicin cream applied four times a day, although it may be used in concentrations of up to 0.075 per cent. Capsaicin is also available in large bandages that can be applied to the back.[30] The most common side effect is a stinging or burning sensation in the area. If possible, wear disposable gloves before applying the cream and be careful not to touch the eye area or apply to broken or irritated skin.

There are many other anti-inflammatory creams available, including boswellia and curcumin. All can be bought in health-food stores and online (see Resources, page 351).

SUMMARY

The best natural anti-inflammatory strategy is to:

- **Eat lots of greens, berries and fruits**, which are high in flavonoids. Have a red onion a day and plenty of olives. Add ginger, pepper-family spices and turmeric liberally to food.
- **Supplement the following** (the lower dose range is best if you are taking a combination of these, whereas the higher dose is better if you wish to test the effects of a single supplement):
    - Curcumin 300–500mg, once or three times a day.
      or boswellia (rich in boswellic acid) 200–400mg, once or twice a day.
      or ashwagandha (providing 1.5 per cent withanolides) 300–500mg, once or twice a day.
    - Quercetin 150–300mg, once or twice a day.
    - Olive extract (providing hydroxytyrosol) 200–400mg, once or twice a day.
    - Hop extract (providing IsoOxygene) 400–800mg a day.

Optional extras:
- Ginger 250–1,000mg, once or twice a day.
- Bromelain 200–400mg, once or twice a day.
- DPA 250mg, three times a day, away from food.
  or DLPA 750mg, three times a day, away from food.

continued

Generally, it is best to take these away from food, for the best absorption; however, the most common side-effect of high-dose use is nausea, in which case either lower the dose or experiment taking it with a small amount of food.

Note If you are in extreme pain you can have these doses three times a day for a short period of time, up to two weeks.

CHAPTER 6

OILING YOUR JOINTS

It's a popular misconception that fish oils lubricate your joints. What they actually do is reduce pain and inflammation by counteracting inflammatory chemicals in the body. They are converted in the body into beneficial anti-inflammatory prostaglandins, which counteract the inflammatory substances that NSAIDs are used to suppress.

It is a story that comes up again and again when comparing drugs and nutritional medicine. All over the body there are chemical accelerators and brakes. We've already seen that COX-1 is involved in producing artery-narrowing thromboxane, whereas COX-2 is part of the pathway that makes the prostacyclin which can reverse that. And the same thing goes on with the chemical chain that produces inflammatory PG2 and anti-inflammatory PG3. But while drugs inevitably create problems when they block part of our system, the food and herbs that we eat don't do that. Otherwise we'd have dismissed them as poisons centuries or millennia ago, and they would never have become part of the human diet.

OMEGA-3S – FATS THAT FIGHT INFLAMMATION

Omega-3 fats are found in oily fish, particularly herring, mackerel, salmon and tuna. They are derived from an essential oil called linolenic acid, which is found in small amounts in some nuts and seeds. The richest source is flax seed, and its oil. Linolenic acid is also found in plankton, which the small fish eat. When larger fish eat small fish they start to concentrate and convert linolenic acid into two complex fats that can be used by the body to produce prostaglandins. These are EPA (eicosapentaenoic acid) and DHA (docosahexaenoic acid). These fats are also concentrated in cod liver oil, but not in the flesh of cod or other white fish.

UNDENIABLE EVIDENCE

There's plenty of research to show conclusively that fish oil supplementation can reduce the inflammation of arthritis. A recent analysis of 17 high-quality trials showed that supplementing omega-3s for three to four months substantially reduced joint pain intensity, morning stiffness and a number of painful and/or tender joints in patients with rheumatoid arthritis or joint pain. NSAID consumption was also reduced by 40 per cent.[31]

In one study 17 patients were given 1.8g of EPA a day. After 12 weeks they had significantly less stiffness and tenderness in their joints. The improvement didn't last when the patients stopped taking the EPA supplements.[32] A further trial on 16 rheumatoid arthritis patients also demonstrated positive results for fish oils over 12 weeks.[33]

In another study, Dr Kremer and his colleagues showed that both the dose of fish oil and the length of time taken have an important effect on the relief experienced.[34] They gave 49 patients with active rheumatoid arthritis either low-dose fish oil (providing 27mg/kg of EPA and 18mg/kg of DHA), high-dose fish oil (providing 54mg/kg EPA and 36mg/kg DHA), or olive oil, under double-blind conditions. They monitored changes over 24 weeks. Improvements in tender joints were most marked in the high-dose fish oil group after 24 weeks, whereas joint swelling decreased significantly after only 12 weeks. Results were best in the high-dose fish oil group. Of the 45 different clinical measures taken to monitor change, 21 improved in the high-dose group, eight in the low-dose group and five in the olive oil group.

The benefits of fish oil were confirmed in a study undertaken in three Danish hospitals.[35] Here, 51 patients with rheumatoid arthritis were given either six fish oil capsules (giving 3.6g of fish oil, equivalent to 1,200mg of EPA) or capsules containing fat with the composition of the normal Danish diet. Although the dosage of EPA was somewhat lower than in earlier trials, the results showed a clear improvement in joint tenderness and morning stiffness in those people who took the fish oil capsules.

Dosage for fish oils

An effective amount to take is the equivalent of 1,000mg of combined omega-3s EPA and DHA a day, which means two to three of most fish oil capsules. DHA converts readily into EPA, although EPA-rich formulas appear most effective.

Cod liver oil

EPA-rich cod liver oil is another possibility. A 2002 study giving cod liver oil to osteoarthritis patients scheduled for knee replacement surgery is a case in point. Half the 31 patients were given two daily capsules of 1,000mg high-strength cod liver oil – rich in the omega-3 fats DHA and EPA – and the other half were given placebo oil capsules for 10–12 weeks. Some 86 per cent of patients with arthritis who took the cod liver oil capsules had no, or markedly reduced, levels of enzymes that cause cartilage damage, as opposed to 26 per cent of those given a placebo.[36] Results also showed a reduction in the inflammatory markers that cause joint pain among those who took the cod liver oil.

Dosage for cod liver oil

Take 1,000mg cod liver oil a day, but check it's high in omega-3.

Fish oils: helping people reduce NSAIDs

All this evidence verifies that large enough amounts of fish oil are anti-inflammatory – probably due to their EPA and DHA content – and may be as effective as NSAID medication in some cases, without the side effects. In fact, one study showed that 39 per cent of rheumatoid arthritis patients were able to reduce their daily NSAIDs by up to 30 per cent when given cod liver oil capsules containing 2.2g of omega-3 fish oils.[37] It is likely that anecdotal reports of cod liver oil helping arthritis stem from the fact that cod liver oil is a very good source of EPA and DHA. Although this is true, the flesh of cod itself has a much lower EPA content than the flesh of carnivorous or oily fish such as mackerel, herring and salmon.

FISH OILS AND ASPIRIN

A word of caution: both fish oil and aspirin thin the blood. They both stop platelets clumping together. The combined use of large amounts of both could therefore lead to a potentially harmful inability of blood to clot, and hence long bleeding times in the case of injuries. It may therefore be prudent not to combine ongoing aspirin and high-dose fish oil use.[38] The same is also true for the more potent blood-thinning drugs such as warfarin and coumadin.

However, it has to be said that you can't have it both ways. If these nutrients do substantially thin the blood, and they do, they are obviously preferable to blood-thinning drugs. So, perhaps the caution should read: 'Do not take warfarin or aspirin if you are supplementing large or combined amounts of omega-3 fish oils.' But since the effect of fish oils is less immediate and less quantified than, for example, warfarin, they shouldn't be used in the short term after a medical crisis. They could be used to reduce the need for anti-coagulant drugs once your condition and your INR (a measure your doctor makes of your blood clotting) are stable.

It's best to discuss all this with your doctor to ensure your INR is monitored as you increase the nutrients, so that the drugs can be reduced accordingly. Unlike drugs, which have many undesirable side effects, the side effects of supplementing omega-3 fish oils is a dramatic reduction in risk of cardiovascular disease, as well as promoting better mood and memory, and less arthritic pain.

Also, if a person has a very poor intake of antioxidant nutrients and is generating a lot of oxidants due to inflammation, these essential fats can themselves be oxidised and may thereby worsen, rather than help, the condition. In these circumstances it is best to restore the oxidant/antioxidant balance by eliminating allergens and adding antioxidant nutrients for a couple of weeks, before adding anti-inflammatory fish oils (the omega-3 fats, EPA and DHA), evening primrose or borage oil (the omega-6 fat, GLA). I explain how to do this in Chapters 9 and 10.

The benefit of healthy eating

The combination of a diet high in antioxidants (found mainly in fruit and vegetables) and high in fish oils has proven highly beneficial. A Danish study, which involved changing the diets of over 100 rheumatoid arthritis sufferers, concluded that those who ate a balanced diet, with plenty of fish and antioxidants, found that their morning stiffness improved, and their swollen joints and pain decreased. Hence, they were able to reduce their medication.[39]

OMEGA-6

In Chapters 3 and 4 we saw how both NSAIDs and steroid drugs reduce inflammation by affecting prostaglandins, but not all prostaglandins trigger pain and inflammation. Prostaglandins are short-lived, hormone-like substances in the body, derived from essential fats found in the diet. Whereas one group of prostaglandins (type 2, shown in Figure 7) encourages inflammation, two other groups of prostaglandins (types 1 and 3) have been shown to reduce inflammation in animals in a variety of studies.[40]

Prostaglandin type 1 (PGE1) is derived from linoleic acid, an omega-6 fat, found in seeds and their oils. Sesame, sunflower and safflower oil are particularly rich sources of these essential fats. The body converts linoleic acid into gamma-

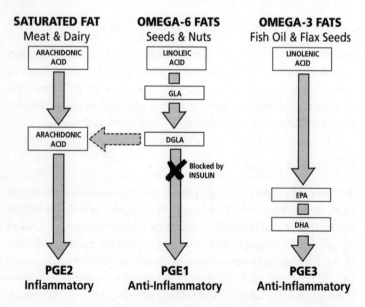

Figure 9 – How prostaglandins control inflammation

linolenic acid (GLA), and then into di-homo gamma-linolenic acid (DGLA), which goes to form prostaglandins, as shown in Figure 9. The conversion step from linoleic acid to gamma-linolenic acid is not so efficient in some people, depending on an enzyme (delta-6-desaturase), which is itself dependent on an adequate supply of vitamin B_6, biotin, zinc and magnesium. Another converting enzyme (delta-5-desaturase) depends on vitamin C and B_3 (niacin).

The ability to convert the essential fats in seeds into anti-inflammatory prostaglandins is also hampered in older people, by a diet high in saturated fat, by alcohol, smoking, sugar and stress. Many people have blood sugar problems, which, in turn, lead to excessive production of the hormone insulin. Insulin also blocks the conversion of linoleic acid into anti-inflammatory prostaglandins, instead leading to the potential formation of pro-inflammatory prostaglandins.

Help from the oils of primrose and borage

For the above reasons GLA, the pre-converted essential fat, which is found particularly in evening primrose oil and borage oil, has been used effectively as an anti-inflammatory nutrient. GLA has been shown to be effective in the treatment of arthritis,[41] arthritis associated with a bacterial infection,[42] and inflammation caused by high uric acid levels (the cause of gout).[43]

Evening primrose oil has proven effective in reducing inflammation and the symptoms of rheumatoid arthritis in three trials. The first trial unwisely stopped NSAID medication abruptly, substituting evening primrose oil for a period of 12 weeks.[44] Although there was no improvement in the arthritis, there was a reduction in inflammation, and only two out of the 17 patients deteriorated, whereas most of them would have been expected to deteriorate coming off NSAID medication. This study suggests that sources of GLA, such as evening primrose oil, may be at least as effective as anti-inflammatory drugs without the same risk of side effects.

In a much longer trial, comparing the effects of essential fats with NSAIDs, the results were definitely positive.[45] Arthritic patients, stable on NSAIDs, were assigned to one of three groups. One received 100 per cent evening primrose oil, one 80 per cent evening primrose oil and 20 per cent fish oil, and the third a placebo. After three months, patients were encouraged to reduce or stop their NSAID medication over the next nine months. At the end of this time, everyone was put on placebos. About 90 per cent of those taking essential fats reported improvement and were able to stop, or at least considerably reduce, the NSAIDs compared with 30 per cent in the placebo group. Almost all who had improved on essential fats regressed when placed on the placebo.

The results from a study at the University of Massachusetts Medical Center, in which people suffering from rheumatoid arthritis were given supplementary GLA, also showed that it was effective in helping to reduce symptoms. For the first six months of the trial, half the volunteers were given GLA, while the other half were given a placebo. After that, all volunteers took GLA for a further six months. Each time, GLA proved to be helpful.[46]

As a natural anti-inflammatory nutrient, GLA, from evening primrose oil and borage, is likely to be at least as effective as NSAIDs in the long run, without side effects or the risk of speeding up the progress of the disease. Whether essential fat supplementation halts or slows down the progress of arthritis is not yet known, but it should reduce inflammation and, consequently, pain.

Dosage for GLA

The amount of GLA required to have this effect is quite high. I recommend 200–300mg of GLA per day, reducing to 150mg after three months if inflammation lessens and symptoms remain stable. Only 9–10 per cent of the oil in evening primrose oil is from GLA so that means initially taking 3,000mg of evening primrose oil, or six 500mg capsules per day. Alternatively, borage oil contains a higher proportion of GLA and you can get single capsules that provide 250mg of GLA. One of these per day is an essential part of an anti-inflammatory strategy. Supplementing GLA has been shown to be more effective when the co-factor vitamins and minerals (vitamin B_6, zinc, B_3 and vitamin C) are also supplied.[47] However, it is important to also supplement an EPA-rich fish oil as well. Not only is omega-3 a more potent anti-inflammatory but also the modern diet is more deficient in omega-3 than omega-6.

The Celadrin story

Talking of fats, there's a special patented blend of fats, called Celadrin that has proved highly effective at reducing arthritic pain in recent double-blind trials compared to a placebo.[48] In one, published in 2002 in the prestigious *Journal of Rheumatology*, 64 patients with chronic knee osteoarthritis were given Celadrin capsules for 68 days. Those taking Celadrin had more flexibility, fewer aches and less pain, and were able to walk longer distances than those in the placebo group. In fact, Celadrin was so effective that the authors concluded that Celadrin might be an alternative to NSAIDs for the treatment of osteoarthritis.[49]

Celadrin contains esterified fats (which means they are stable and do not react with oxygen). These fats have pronounced anti-inflammatory effects, which is very important to prevent further tissue and joint damage. Like so many natural remedies, Celadrin seems to work on many

continued

different fronts. It works to stop inflammation (by inhibiting COX-2 and 5-LOX) although it does not appear to rebuild joints, unlike nutrients such as glucosamine, which repairs and regenerates cartilage (discussed in Chapter 16). It is available in capsules, tablets, soft gels or as a cream (see Anti-inflammatory Gels and Creams, page 55).

Although Celadrin is fairly new to the market, many people have reported enormous benefits.

Case Study: Sue and Ann

Having suffered from shoulder problems for 13 years, Sue found herself suffering from the most severe bout of pain. Here's what she had to say:

'For four weeks, every night brought the most incredible pain in both shoulders, causing me to wake four or five times in the night. At this time I became desperate! I was no longer able to deal well with stressful situations due to lack of sleep. An MRI scan revealed that I had bursitis in both shoulders, plus some intra-tendonous tearing of my left shoulder. Unhappy with the potential side effects of my medication and their ineffectiveness, I was advised to take Celadrin. On the Saturday morning I started taking them three times a day, as suggested. Monday night I slept pain-free for the first time in two months. Today I am still pain-free. I have told just about everyone I know how amazing this product is.'

Ann, who has been taking Celadrin for 9 months, used to suffer from aches and pains in her neck, shoulders, elbows and knees but has noticed a definite improvement since taking Celadrin:

'Whilst I still suffer, on occasions, from some pain, I simply double the dosage for a few days and I can feel the difference.

I can sincerely say that, since taking Celadrin, my problems have been significantly less.'

Others have found that a combination of Celadrin and glu–cosamine is very effective at reducing pain and increasing movement in their joints.

SUMMARY

- **Increase your intake of omega-3 fats** by eating oily fish, such as herring, mackerel or salmon two to three times a week.
- **Eat nuts and seeds, and their oils** – among the best are flax, sesame, sunflower and pumpkin.
- **Supplement** between 1,000mg and 2,000mg of EPA; and 200–600mg of DHA a day.
- **If taking aspirin**, or other blood-thinning medication such as warfarin, do not take high-dose fish oils without consulting your doctor.
- **Take an appropriate dose of GLA** (omega-6): 200–300mg per day, reducing to 150mg after three months if inflammation lessens and symptoms remain stable. Since evening primrose oil (EPO) contains about 10 per cent GLA, this means supplementing 2,000–3,000mg (usually 4–6 500mg capsules) of EPO initially, reducing to 1,500mg (3 500mg capsules).
- **Ensure that your diet is high in antioxidant nutrients** by eating plenty of fruits and vegetables. Otherwise the essential fats themselves may become oxidised (see Chapter 10).

CHAPTER 7

SUGAR – THE SWEET TRUTH

Keeping your blood sugar level even is critical in order to combat arthritis and maintain overall health. Insulin, the major hormone released by your body to control blood sugar, stimulates the production and assembly of proteoglycans (the cartilage-building compound) into cartilage.[50] Diabetics, who are either deficient in insulin or insensitive to it (known as 'insulin resistance'), have more severe arthritis than non-diabetic arthritis sufferers.[51]

This is because one of the main causes of inflammation and damage to joints is glycation, which means damage caused by sugar. Glycation is inflammation caused by glucose imbalance and insulin resistance. Glucose can damage joints in the same way that it damages arteries, which is why there is a strong link between diabetes and arthritis. Although ordinarily the adrenal hormone cortisol – the body's best anti-inflammatory agent – can handle such problems, out-of-control blood sugar results in adrenal exhaustion. This is because blood sugar lows promote the excessive release of adrenal hormones, effectively turning you into a hungry hunter for food, or another sugar fix or a stimulant pick-me-up, both of which contribute to worsening blood sugar control and increasing inflammation. So it's far better to keep your blood sugar balanced to prevent inflammation in the first place.

Having an uneven blood sugar level also upsets calcium balance and is clearly a risk factor for arthritis. In addition, keeping your blood sugar balanced is probably the most important factor in weight control.

HOW BLOOD GLUCOSE LEVELS ALSO AFFECT WEIGHT GAIN

The level of glucose in your blood largely determines your appetite. When the level drops, you feel hungry. The glucose in your bloodstream is available to body cells to make energy. When the levels are too high, the body converts the excess to glycogen (which is a short-term fuel mainly stored in the liver and muscle cells) or fat, our long-term energy reserve. When the levels are too low, we experience a whole host of symptoms, including fatigue, poor concentration, irritability, nervousness, depression, excessive thirst, sweating, headaches and digestive problems. An estimated three in every ten people have glucose intolerance (an inability to keep an even blood sugar level). Their blood sugar level may go up too high and then drop too low. The result, over the years, is that they become increasingly fat and lethargic, which can also lead to joint problems later on. On the other hand, if you can control your blood sugar levels, the result is even weight and constant energy.

Questionnaire: check your glucose tolerance

Tick the box for yes or no.

	Yes	No
1 Are you rarely wide awake within 20 minutes of rising?	☐	☐
2 Do you need tea, coffee, a cigarette or something sweet to get you going in the morning?	☐	☐

3 Do you really like sweet foods?   ☐ ☐

4 Do you crave bread, cereal, popcorn
   or pasta?   ☐ ☐

5 Do you feel that you 'need' an alcoholic
   drink on most days?   ☐ ☐

6 Are you overweight and unable to shift
   the extra pounds?   ☐ ☐

7 Do you often have energy slumps
   throughout the day or after meals?   ☐ ☐

8 Do you have mood swings or difficulty
   concentrating?   ☐ ☐

9 Do you get dizzy or irritable if you go
   six hours without food?   ☐ ☐

10 Do you often find you over-react to stress?   ☐ ☐

11 Do you often get irritable, angry or
   aggressive unexpectedly?   ☐ ☐

12 Is your energy level now lower than it
   used to be?   ☐ ☐

13 Do you ever lie about how much sweet
   food you have eaten?   ☐ ☐

14 Do you ever keep a supply of sweet food
   close to hand?   ☐ ☐

15 Do you feel you could never give up bread? ☐ ☐

Score 1 for each 'yes' answer, then add up
your score.

Total score: ☐

Score

If you answered 'yes' to eight or more of the questions above there's a strong possibility that your body is having difficulty keeping your blood sugar level even.

FAST-RELEASE AND SLOW-RELEASE FOODS

So what makes your blood sugar level unbalanced? Obviously, eating too much sugar and sweet foods. However, the kinds of food that have the greatest effect are not always the ones you might expect.

Eat low-GL foods

The measure of what a food does to your blood sugar is known as the glycemic load (GL). Neither protein nor fat (for example, meat, fish, cheese or eggs) have any substantial effect on your blood sugar balance, so we are talking here about sugary or carbohydrate-rich foods.

The sugars and starches in foods with a high GL (refined carbohydrates, such as white bread, sweets and biscuits) are broken down and absorbed quickly into the bloodstream, making your blood glucose levels soar. You are likely to experience an increase in energy followed by an energy crash when your blood sugar drops, and you will probably reach for something sweet in order to relieve the symptoms of low blood sugar. Meanwhile, the sugars and starches in foods with a low-GL (complex carbohydrates such as wholegrains, vegetables, beans or lentils, or simpler carbohydrates such as fruit) take longer to digest than refined carbohydrates. As a result, the glucose released from these foods trickles slowly into the bloodstream. This means that it's used for energy rather than being stored, leaving blood glucose levels on an even keel, and preventing dramatic changes in your mood, behaviour and energy.

The carbs that keep blood sugar even

The chart below gives the GL score of an average serving of a range of common foods. Foods with a GL of less than 10 (**in bold**) are good and should be the staple foods of your diet. A GL of 11–14 (in regular type) can be eaten in moderation. A GL higher than 15 (*in italics*) should be avoided.

Glycemic load of common foods

Food	Serving size in grams	Serving	GLs per serving
Bakery products			
low-carb muffin	**60**	**1 muffin**	**5**
muffin – apple, made without sugar	**60**	**1 muffin**	**9**
muffin – apple, made with sugar	60	1 muffin	13
crumpet	50	1 crumpet	13
croissant	*57*	*1 croissant*	*17*
doughnut, plain	*47*	*1 doughnut*	*17*
sponge cake, plain	*63*	*1 slice*	*17*
Breads			
wholemeal rye or pumpernickel-style rye bread	**20**	**1 thin slice**	**5**
wheat tortilla (Mexican)	**30**	**1 tortilla**	**5**
wholemeal wheat-flour bread	**30**	**1 thick slice**	**9**
pitta bread, white	**30**	**1 pitta bread**	**10**
baguette, white, plain	*30*	*⅓ baton*	*15*
bagel, white	*70*	*1 bagel*	*25*
Crispbreads and crackers			
rough oatcakes (Nairn's)	**10**	**1 oatcake**	**2**
fine oatcakes (Nairn's)	**9**	**1 oatcake**	**3**
cream cracker	25	2 biscuits	11

Food	Serving size in grams	Serving	GLs per serving
rye crispbread	25	2 biscuits	11
water cracker	*25*	*3 biscuits*	*17*
puffed rice cakes	*25*	*3 biscuits*	*17*
Dairy products and alternatives			
yogurt (plain, no sugar)	**200**	**1 small pot**	**3**
non-fat yogurt (plain, no sugar)	**200**	**1 small pot**	**3**
soya yogurt (Provamel)	**200**	**1 large bowl**	**7**
soya milk (no sugar)	**250 ml**	**1 glass**	**7**
low-fat yogurt, fruit, sugar (Ski)	**150**	**1 small pot**	**7.5**
Fruit and fruit products			
blackberries, raw	**120**	**1 medium bowl**	**1**
blueberries, raw	**120**	**1 medium bowl**	**1**
raspberries, raw	**120**	**1 medium bowl**	**1**
strawberries, raw	**120**	**1 medium bowl**	**1**
cherries, raw	**120**	**1 medium bowl**	**3**
grapefruit, raw	**120**	**½ medium**	**3**
pear, raw	**120**	**1 medium**	**4**
melon/cantaloupe, raw	**120**	**½ small**	**4**
watermelon, raw	**120**	**1 medium slice**	**4**
apricots, raw	**120**	**4**	**5**
oranges, raw	**120**	**1 large**	**5**
plum, raw	**120**	**4**	**5**
apple, raw	**120**	**1 small**	**6**
kiwi fruit, raw	**120**	**1**	**6**
pineapple, raw	**120**	**1 medium slice**	**7**
grapes, raw	**120**	**16**	**8**
mango, raw	**120**	**1½ slices**	**8**
apricots, dried	**60**	**6**	**9**
fruit cocktail, canned (Del Monte)	**120**	**1 small can**	**9**
papaya, raw	**120**	**½ small papaya**	**10**

Food	Serving size in grams	Serving	GLs per serving
prunes, pitted	**60**	**6**	**10**
apple, dried	**60**	**6 rings**	**10**
banana, raw	120	1 small	12
apricots, canned in light syrup	120	1 small can	12
lychees, canned in syrup and drained	120	1 small can	16
figs, dried, tenderised (Dessert Maid)	60	3	16
sultanas	60	30	25
raisins	60	30	28
dates, dried	60	8	42
Jams/spreads			
pumpkin seed butter	**16**	**1 tbsp**	**1**
peanut butter (no sugar)	**16**	**1 tbsp**	**1**
blueberry spread (no sugar)	**10**	**2 tsp**	**1**
orange marmalade	**10**	**2 tsp**	**3**
strawberry jam	**10**	**2 tsp**	**3**
Snack foods (savoury)			
eggs (boiled)	**–**	**2 medium**	**0**
cottage cheese	**120**	**½ medium tub**	**2**
hummus	**200**	**1 small tub**	**6**
olives, in brine	**50**	**7**	**1**
peanuts	**50**	**2 medium handfuls**	**1**
cashew nuts, salted	**50**	**2 medium handfuls**	**3**
potato crisps, plain, salted	**30**	**1 small packet**	**7**
popcorn, salted	**25**	**1 small packet**	**10**
pretzels, oven-baked, traditional wheat flavour	30	15	16
corn chips, plain, salted	50	18	17
Snack foods (sweet)			
Fruitus apple cereal bar	**35**	**1**	**5**

Food	Serving size in grams	Serving	GLs per serving
Euroviva Rebar fruit and veg bar	**50**	**1**	**8**
muesli bar with dried fruit	30	1	13
chocolate bar, milk, plain (Mars/Cadbury/Nestlé)	50	1	14
Twix biscuit and caramel bar (Mars)	60	*1 bar (2 fingers)*	*17*
Snickers bar (Mars)	60	*1*	*19*
Polos, peppermint sweets (Nestlé)	30	*16*	*21*
Jelly beans, assorted colours	30	*9*	*22*
Kellogg's Pop-Tarts, double choc	50	*1*	*24*
Mars Bar	60	*1*	*26*

A comprehensive list of the GL values of foods is also available online at www.holforddiet.com.

Healthy snack options

Try these alternatives:

Instead of crisps have oatcakes, pumpkin seeds, roasted snack mix or plain popcorn.

Instead of biscuits have sweet oatcake biscuits (such as Nairn's) or fruit or nut bars (such as Fruitus bar by Lyme Regis Foods).

Instead of sweets and chocolate have fresh fruit (apple, pear, peach, plum, berries), dried fruits such as apricots (these are a concentrated source of natural sugars, so eat in moderation).

Instead of sugar (in drinks and home baking) have xylitol (it tastes just like sugar but doesn't upset blood sugar balance or cause tooth decay).

continued

Instead of sweetened drinks drink water, fruity/herbal teas, diluted fruit juice (gradually increase the amount of water to let your taste buds adjust), diluted apple and blackcurrant concentrate, such as Meridian or cherry concentrate such as Cherry Active.

Stimulants, stress and the sugar response

Alcohol, a chemical cousin of sugar, also upsets blood sugar levels. So do stimulants, such as tea, coffee, cola drinks and cigarettes. These substances, like stress itself, stimulate the release of adrenalin and other hormones that initiate the 'fight or flight' response. This prepares the body for action, by releasing sugar stores and raising blood sugar levels, to give our muscles and brains a boost of energy. Unlike our ancestors, whose main stresses required a physical response (like climbing up a tree to avoid being eaten for dinner), 20th-century stress is mainly mental or emotional. It still provokes the same response though, so the body has to cope with the excess of blood sugar by releasing yet more hormones to take the glucose out of circulation. The combination of too much sugar, stimulants and prolonged stress taxes the body and results in an inability to control blood sugar levels, which, if severe enough, can develop into diabetes.

GETTING OUT OF THE CYCLE

The only way out of this vicious circle is to reduce or avoid all forms of concentrated sweetness, tea, coffee, alcohol and cigarettes, and start eating foods that help to keep your blood sugar level even. The best foods are all kinds of beans, peas and lentils, oats and wholegrains. These foods are high in complex carbohydrates and contain special factors that help release their sugar content gradually. They are also high in fibre, which helps normalise blood sugar levels.

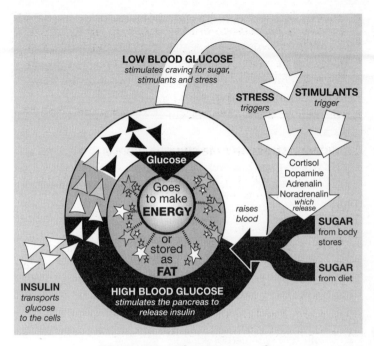

Figure 10 – The sugar cycle

Eating sugar increases blood glucose levels. The body releases insulin into the blood to help escort glucose out and into body cells, to make energy or convert into fat. The result is low blood glucose. Either stress, causing more adrenalin, or induced stress, caused by consuming a stimulant such as caffeine, which raises adrenal hormones, causes breakdown of stores of sugar in the liver and muscles, called glycogen, which raises blood sugar levels. Low blood glucose causes stress or cravings for either something sweet or a stimulant.

Eat protein with carbohydrate

The more fibre and protein you include with any meal or snack, the slower the release of the carbohydrates, which is good for blood-glucose balance. So, combining protein-rich foods with high-fibre carbohydrates is an excellent rule of thumb.

Ways to combine carbohydrates and protein:

- Eat unsalted seeds or nuts with a whole fruit snack.
- Add seeds or nuts to carbohydrate-based breakfast cereals.
- Top wholemeal toast with eggs, baked beans or nut butter.
- Serve salmon or chicken with brown basmati rice.
- Add kidney beans to pasta sauce served over wholemeal pasta.
- Put cottage cheese on oatcakes, or hummus on pumpernickel-style whole-grain rye bread.
- Make sandwiches with sugar-free peanut butter and wholemeal bread.

SUMMARY

There are three golden rules to mastering your blood sugar balance:

1 Eat low-GL foods.
2 Eat protein with carbohydrate.
3 Graze, don't gorge – eat little and often.

CHAPTER 8

DETOX YOUR JOINTS

There is one diet that has consistently worked for sufferers of arthritis, particularly rheumatoid arthritis, and that is – not eating. Fasts, or modified fasts with fruit and vegetable juices, have proven to be possibly the most successful dietary strategy to date, reducing most symptoms (subjectively and objectively) within days.[52] However, there is a risk of losing weight by this strategy, so if you're not overweight, it might not be the best thing to do.

What is it about fasting that produces such good results? The most likely explanation is that a food or drink is aggravating arthritis. There are many possible areas currently being investigated to explain why many arthritis sufferers get better when avoiding certain foods or drinks. These include food allergies or intolerances, increased intestinal permeability (known as 'leaky gut'), pathogens in the gut, poor liver detox-ification and oxidative stress.[53] Oxidative stress is caused by too many molecules in the body known as 'free radicals', which I explain in Chapter 10.

These can be seen as a vicious circle of problems, starting in the digestive tract and setting the scene for inflammation and arthritis, as shown in Figure 11.

This illustration shows just how most states of ill health develop: they knock your body's ecosystem out of balance. Eating the wrong foods, or foods you are allergic to, or if you

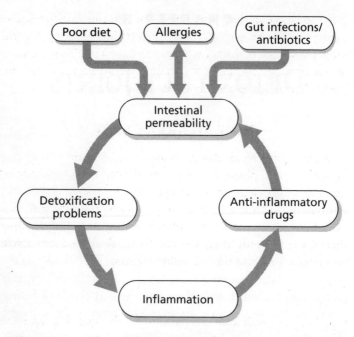

Figure 11 – The vicious circle of toxic overload and inflammation

(Adapted with the permission of Helen Kimber, Nutri Ltd.)

become infected with harmful bacteria, fungi or other un-desirable microbes, these can all damage your digestive tract, often resulting in increased intestinal permeability, or leaky gut. This means that incompletely digested food and toxic matter can enter your system, stimulating allergic responses and taxing your body's natural ability to detoxify. Overload leads to oxidative stress, with more free-radical activity. This causes inflammation, which is then treated by drugs that fur-ther damage the digestive tract and increase intestinal perme-ability, making matters worse. It also explains a key dynamic of many drugs. They may make you feel better instantly, but they don't solve the underlying disease – and in this case they make matters worse. So you've got to keep taking the drug, but the longer you take it, the more side effects you get. This scenario, in one form or another, is exceedingly common among people with arthritis, especially rheumatoid arthritis.

HOW TO BREAK FREE

The alternative to all this is an approach that aims to restore health to your physical ecosystem. If you visit a nutritional therapist, each element of the cycle can be tested, from 'leaky gut syndrome' to whether or not your body is reacting allergically to foods by producing antibodies. It's hard science rather than throwing pills at symptoms. To break the vicious circle, you need to address the following factors:

- diet
- allergies
- pathogens (undesirable organisms in the gut that upset its balance)
- intestinal permeability, often known as 'leaky gut'
- detoxification problems (when your body is unable to detoxify efficiently)
- free radicals

DIET

A poor diet leads to an unhealthy digestive tract. It's particularly important to avoid or reduce alcohol and wheat, both of which act as irritants. A lack of nutrients means the body won't digest foods properly. Zinc is especially important in this regard. Vitamin A is also needed for a healthy intestinal tract. Too much fried food, coupled with a lack of antioxidants from fruit and vegetables, can cause oxidative damage to the digestive tract. All these factors increase the chances of developing idiosyncratic reactions to foods. Part 5 explains what you need to eat for optimal health.

ALLERGIES

An allergy is an unusual response to a substance, whether drunk, eaten, inhaled or applied to the skin, which causes a reaction in the body's immune system – a process that causes inflammation. Because the whole process of inflammation is part of the body's immune reaction, and since there is so much evidence of abnormal immune responses in arthritis sufferers, an allergic reaction could easily encourage symptoms of arthritis. Food intolerance is a term applied to foods that seem to make matters worse, but for which there is no clear allergic response. We do not yet know how some substances aggravate arthritis, but many foods are known to cause symptoms of arthritis in susceptible people. The next chapter explains how to investigate whether or not you are susceptible to specific food allergies or intolerances, and how to eliminate the culprits.

THE IMPORTANCE OF BALANCE IN THE GUT

The undesirable organisms that reside in the guts of many people are called pathogens. We all have approximately 1.3kg (3lb) of about 300 different strains of bacteria living within our gut. Some can be classified as good and others as bad. However, the potentially 'bad' guys are not a hindrance as long as there are enough of the good guys around. These bacteria help us to digest food and fight off bad bacteria that enter the body, and they even make some vitamins. But the presence of the wrong kind of bacteria can cause ill health – especially if the gut wall is permeable and they enter the bloodstream. In animal studies, overgrowth of undesirable gut bacteria has been shown to induce the inflammatory symptoms of arthritis, increasing pain levels.[54] This connection between poor diet and dysbiosis (the official term for having an unhealthy balance of micro-organisms in the digestive tract) is being widely researched, and it is certainly plausible that dysbiosis is a potential contributor to arthritis, especially rheumatoid arthritis.[55]

Another common pathogen in the gut is *Candida albicans*. This is a yeast-like organism, which, if it becomes established, sends roots into the gut wall and increases gut permeability. Sounds nasty, doesn't it? *Candida albicans* infection is increasingly common, and, once again, eating certain foods, particularly sugary ones, will aggravate this condition.

Based on the current evidence, it is unlikely that the presence of a pathogen such as *Candida albicans* is a common contributory cause of arthritis, but it is worth bearing in mind, especially if you have digestive problems. Pathogens often thrive in an unhealthy digestive tract. A nutritional therapist can recommend tests, if this is something that concerns you (see Resources, page 348).

THE PROBLEMS OF A LEAKY GUT

Normally, the inner lining of your small intestine serves as a highly selective barrier against your internal environment, preventing the entry of potentially harmful toxins, microbes and incompletely digested foods from the gut into blood circulation in much the same way that a bouncer keeps the riff-raff out of an exclusive club. At the same time, this lining selectively allows the important vitamins, minerals, amino acids, essential fats, simple sugars and other nutrients to pass into the body via the bloodstream. These are the breakdown products of properly digested food and only these should get through into your bloodstream.

Poor digestion and food sensitivity often go together. The reason is that if you eat foods you are unknowingly allergic to or that you don't digest very well – for example, gluten in wheat – or drink alcohol, or take painkillers frequently, they can irritate your digestive tract. This can add up to a pretty hefty problem, as the surface area of your digestive tract is the size of a small football pitch. Gradually, if you continue to consume the irritants, your gut will become less healthy and more leaky.

How a leaky gut affects your immune system

This condition, known as gastrointestinal permeability, has been the focus of some 1,500 studies. Food particles can enter the blood, and the immune system is then exposed to proteins that are not on the guest list, so to speak, triggering a reaction in the immune system. This is the source of most food allergies (see Chapter 9). The immune army goes on red alert to deal with the unwelcome guests, thereby encouraging immune reactions that also take place in the joints, causing inflammation. If the gut wall is excessively permeable, eating virtually any diet may make symptoms worse. Gut permeability can be caused by food allergies in the gut, which weaken the wall of the digestive tract, by the presence of undesirable organisms like bacteria or the fungus *Candida albicans*, or by the lack of key nutrients, such as vitamins A and C, and zinc, which are needed to keep the wall of the digestive tract strong and healthy. Over time the leakiness leads to more inflammation and, eventually, weaker immunity. So you might develop irritable bowel syndrome, asthma, eczema or arthritis (all of which are inflammatory diseases that have been strongly linked to food allergy), or become more prone to infections. If you are given a non-steroidal painkiller, such as aspirin or ibuprofen, or a course of antibiotics, this further irritates the gut and makes it more permeable.

Intestinal permeability varies from person to person. Those with inflammatory arthritis (and especially rheumatoid arthritis sufferers) often have increased gut permeability, which may be made worse by NSAID medication.[56]

How can you repair a leaky gut?

Increased intestinal permeability can be measured by a simple, non-invasive test that can be done at home. A test kit can be obtained from a nutritional therapist (see Resources, page 348). If the results indicate increased permeability, the therapist will advise you to follow a specific diet that is low in gluten (among other foods), and recommend supplements that will help to heal the digestive tract. These include the amino acid glutamine, plus antioxidants A, C and zinc. The ideal intake of glutamine for healing a leaky gut is 5g a day.

WHEN YOUR BODY HAS DETOXIFICATION PROBLEMS

Instead of thinking of certain substances as 'bad' for you, or provoking allergies, think of them as being more than your body can adapt to. It's as if your metabolism is a fire. The fire generates smoke, which must be removed. Energy from the sun is stored in plants. When we eat the plants, our metabolic 'fire' burns this energy 24 hours a day, generating plenty of smoke. The toxins that enter the body from food and from its breakdown in the digestive tract, as well as the 'exhaust' we generate from burning food all have to be detoxified. These detoxification processes occur mainly in the liver but also in the digestive tract and, to some extent, in most cells. Many people with inflammatory conditions such as arthritis, however, have poor detoxification abilities.

HOW THE LIVER WORKS

The way the liver detoxifies the 'smoke' can be split into two stages (see Figure 12 on page 89). The first, known as Phase 1, is similar to getting your household rubbish ready for collection. It doesn't actually eliminate anything, but just prepares it for elimination, making it easier to pick up. Fat-soluble toxins, for example, become more soluble. Phase 1 is carried out by a series of enzymes called P-450 enzymes. The more toxins you're exposed to, the faster these enzymes must work to pile up rubbish ready for collection. Often, the substances created by the P-450 enzyme reactions are actually more toxic than before. For example, many are oxidised, generating harmful oxidants (also known as free radicals).

Phase 1

The function of P-450 enzymes depends on a long list of nutrients, including vitamins C and E, beta-carotene, glutathione, N-acetyl cysteine, coenzyme Q10 and selenium. Often a person who has a high exposure to toxins (perhaps due to diet and lifestyle factors or digestive problems) has a 'revved-up' Phase 1, which is used to working hard and fast to get these toxins ready for collection. Substances that 'rev up' Phase 1 include caffeine, alcohol, dioxins, cigarette smoke, exhaust fumes, high-protein diets, organophosphate fertilisers, paint fumes, saturated fat, steroid hormones and charcoal-barbecued meat.

Phase 2

The second phase, known as Phase 2, is more about building up than breaking down. According to Dr Sidney Baker, an expert in the chemistry of detoxification, around 80 per cent of all the 'building' that the body does is for the purposes of detoxification. The end products of Phase 1 are transformed by 'sticking' things on to them in a process called conjugation. Some toxins have glutathione stuck to them (this is called

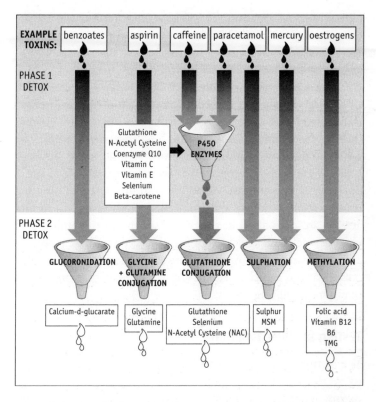

Figure 12 – The key detox nutrients your liver needs

glutathione conjugation). This is how we detoxify paracetamol (acetaminophen), for example. In cases of overdose, a person is given glutathione to mop up the highly destructive toxins generated by Phase 1 detoxification of this drug.

Other toxins have sulphur stuck to them in a process called sulphation. This is the fate of many steroid hormones, neuro-transmitters and, once again, paracetamol. The sulphur comes directly from food. Garlic, onions and eggs, for example, are good sources of sulphur-containing amino acids such as methionine and cysteine – so if you lack these you've got a problem. Others have carbon compounds, called methyl groups, stuck to them – this is called methylation. Lead and arsenic are detoxified in this way. Aspirin has the amino acid glycine stuck to it (glycine conjugation). When these pathways are overloaded, the body can use another, known as glu-curonidation, which is the primary route for breaking down many tranquillising drugs.

Testing for liver function

When these biochemical pathways don't work properly, due to overload or a lack of nutrients, the body generates harmful toxins. Standard tests for liver function involve measuring lev-els of key enzymes AST and ALT. If they are raised, it means your liver is struggling. This indicates a chronic problem but, although it is useful in pinpointing that a problem exists, it doesn't really identify the best way to help recovery.

A Comprehensive Detoxification Profile provides a more advanced and detailed indication of liver function, and can pick up imbalances before they develop into chronic health problems. This is a non-invasive test that involves ingesting a measured amount of caffeine, aspirin and paracetamol and then analysing certain chemicals that appear in the urine. How these substances are dealt with, and what they turn into, helps determine which pathways are working and which ones aren't. If one pathway is under-functioning, another may be over-functioning to help cope with the load. Researchers at the University of Birmingham tested detoxification potential in patients with rheumatoid arthritis by challenging the liver with low-dose paracetamol and measuring liver function. They found that these patients were not able to detoxify paracetamol well; this meant that they were particularly susceptible to the toxic effects of the drug.[57]

HOW TO RESTORE AND MAINTAIN OPTIMAL LIVER FUNCTION

The good news is that, with the right nutrients, you can restore optimal liver function; and, with a good diet, lifestyle and the right supplements, you can maintain liver function at optimal levels. For those with chronic health problems, especially conditions involving chronic fatigue, allergies or chemical sensitivities, or digestive disorders, it is well worth seeing a nutritional therapist and having the necessary tests. They can help identify the sources of toxic overload and indicate how to eliminate them, as well as giving the right balance of nutrients to get the liver's log-jam moving again.

Prevention, however, is always better than cure. If you are basically healthy and want to promote and maintain optimal liver function, the best advice is to cut down on your intake of toxic substances, eat an optimal diet and take a balanced range of supplements. Key foods are fruits and vegetables, especially those rich in glucosinolates, which help the liver to detoxify. These include cabbage, broccoli, Brussels sprouts and kale. Artichokes and turmeric also aid liver function.

Supplements for liver function

Start with a high-strength multivitamin and mineral, additional antioxidant nutrients and at least 2,000mg of vitamin C.

Another vitamin that specifically helps to speed up detoxification of the body is vitamin B_3 in the form of niacin. Niacin is different from niacinamide, which is recommended in Chapter 11 for increasing joint flexibility. The niacin form of vitamin B_3 is a 'vasodilator', which means that it dilates or enlarges the tiny blood vessels, called capillaries, which deliver nutrients to cells and collect toxins. This helps them to nourish and detoxify cells. Niacin is used to help eliminate drug residues in the body and has proven highly effective in helping drug addicts to withdraw and poison victims to recover.

Niacin consequently causes a temporary 'blush'. Your body goes red, a bit like if you have mild sunburn; and you may get hot and a little itchy. This usually takes up to 15 minutes to happen, lasts for up to 30 minutes and is not harmful, although some people find it unpleasant. In fact, it is very beneficial and illustrates just how potent nutrients are. Experiment with taking 100mg each day on an empty stomach. (Make sure you buy niacin, not niacinamide.) Since you can get a little cold after a niacin blush this is a great time to have a hot bath. It's best to take niacin in the evening, in the comfort of your own home – not at work or in a potentially stressful environment. Initially your joints may ache more during the blush, and then show improvement. The after-effects of niacin are very calming and may also help to give you a good night's sleep.

Some supplement companies also produce specific nutrient combinations designed to support liver function. Nutrients that can specifically help the liver to function are choline, methionine, liver extract and the herbs milk thistle (which contains silymarin) and dandelion root. Also very helpful is the key antioxidant glutathione, which is recycled by anthocyanidins found in blue/red berries.

FREE RADICALS

One of the most prevalent toxins we have to deal with are oxidants, or free radicals. These are the by-products of breaking down carbohydrate to release energy. We generate these in our bodies but we also take in extra ones from burnt and fried food, smoke, exhaust fumes and other pollutants. When the liver detoxification process isn't working correctly, it also generates excess oxidants. So too does the immune system if it is activated; for example, in the state of inflammation. These oxidants make inflammation worse and are capable of damaging joints and surrounding tissue. Therefore, it is common to find that people with inflammatory arthritis are in a state of 'oxidative stress'.

How to fight free radicals

The antidote to these oxidants is to increase your intake of antioxidants – especially nutrients capable of disarming these free radicals. They include vitamins A, C and E, the minerals selenium and zinc, plus co-enzyme Q_{10}, glutathione and flavonoids (found in foods such as quercetin and curcumin). All the above are discussed in Chapter 10, which explains the wealth of evidence in favour of ensuring an optimal intake of key antioxidant nutrients to reverse the arthritic process and reduce pain and inflammation. Suffice it to say that a key part of an anti-arthritis diet is to cut down your intake of toxins and oxidants, and increase your intake of antioxidants, which are most abundant in fresh fruit and vegetables, especially carrots, tomatoes, green peppers, watercress, berries, beetroot and red grapes.

SUMMARY

There are many ways to become caught up in a vicious circle of toxic overload, which is often a key trigger for arthritis. The following tips will help you decrease your intake of toxins and increase your body's detoxification capacity:

- **Minimise your intake of toxins**: alcohol, caffeine, cigarettes, sugar, fried foods, saturated fat, pesticides, exhaust fumes and medications.
- **Increase your intake of all fruits and vegetables** especially those rich in antioxidants (such as carrots, tomatoes, green peppers, watercress); anthocyanidins (such as berries, beetroot, grapes); and glucosinolates (such as cabbage, broccoli, Brussels sprouts, kale). Also include plenty of onions and garlic.
- **Avoid red meat and dairy products** Eat carnivorous fish in place of meat; cold-pressed seeds and seed oils instead of butter; and drink plenty of purified water.
- **Avoid foods you are allergic to** Chapter 9 will tell you how to find out which these are.
- **Test for gut permeability (leaky gut) or liver detoxification** – if you suspect you are suffering from either problem, consult a nutritional therapist, who will be able to advise you and recommend suitable tests.
- **Take specific nutrient combinations**, specifically those designed to support liver function, including choline, methionine, glutathione, milk thistle, artichoke and dandelion root.
- **Consult a nutritional therapist** Once other factors have been eliminated (such as allergies, liver detoxification problems or dysbiosis), consult a nutritional therapist for advice on how to 'repair' your gut using nutrients such as glutamine, vitamins A and C, and zinc.

CHAPTER 9

WHY FOOD ALLERGIES PROMOTE INFLAMMATION

Allergies are much more common than you think. In fact, almost one in every three people suffers from allergies – whether to pollen, cats, house dust, foods, drugs or chemicals.[58] Among arthritis sufferers, the incidence of allergies is likely to be much higher.

With rheumatoid arthritis, as with other autoimmune diseases like lupus or type-1 diabetes, it's well worth suspecting food allergy as the trigger – especially gluten, soya and/or dairy sensitivities. One theory about why food allergy could trigger autoimmune conditions is that the immune system could become sensitive to a food protein, such as soya or milk protein, and wrongly 'cross-react' to tissue in the body (which is, of course, largely protein). My 25 years of clinical experience has taught me that rheumatoid arthritis is occasionally caused and often provoked by food allergy, and that most rheumatoid arthritis sufferers under the age of 70 respond well to food allergy elimination, together with an optimum-nutrition diet and supplements.

Although an allergy-free diet doesn't help everybody, studies do show that some people experience great benefits. One study in 1992 showed that 9 per cent of a group of rheumatoid arthritis patients improved when put on an allergy-free diet, and worsened when taken off it. To make sure these results were real, six of these patients were reintroduced to small amounts of either non-allergic foods or allergic foods, without knowing which they were taking. Four got noticeably worse on the allergy food, not the placebo.[59]

Although food allergy isn't the only factor contributing to arthritis, I recommend exploring it if you do suffer from arthritis or joint aches and pains. Some people benefit tremendously from testing for and then avoiding identified food allergens.

Case Study: John

John developed arthritis in his toes, fingers, ankles and knees at the age of 23. When he turned 40, he couldn't sleep at night from the pain and had to go upstairs on his hands and knees. Walking just 100 metres was painful. He used to have to think carefully where to park the car when going out so as not to have to walk too far. Holidays were awful. He saw consultants, read books and took lots of medication, but although the medication controlled the pain it had its own side effects: stomach pain and depression. Sometimes John had steroid injections to quell the pain, but it would return later in the day.

Then John heard about food allergy testing. Although his doctor actively discouraged testing of that type, saying that there was 'absolutely no clinical evidence' that altering the diet would improve such a condition, John went ahead and discovered he was allergic to three different foods. He was shocked to discover that the main one was white fish, as everyone had been saying he should cut out red meat and eat much more fish. Egg white and tea were the other two (John remembered sitting and drinking a cup of tea when opening his results!).

John cut them all out. Gradually the number of painkillers he needed lessened and eventually he stopped taking them altogether. In his own words:

> 'Life is now pain- and tablet-free and I have complete mobility. I am amazed at the difference in my quality of life simply by making such simple adjustments.'

John reacted to white fish, egg white and tea. Some people react to wheat or milk, others to vegetables in the nightshade family (aubergine, tomatoes, potatoes and peppers). It's worth being tested to find out if you have an allergy. (For details on food allergy tests, see Resources, page 348).

WHAT IS AN ALLERGY?

To answer this question, you need to know a bit about your immune system. Inside your body is an army of immune cells on a 24-hour search-and-destroy mission. When they find an invader, such as a virus, they destroy it. The main way they capture their prey is by producing a tailor-made 'straitjacket' – an antibody – to fit a particular invader. This is how vaccination works: the polio vaccine exposes your body to the polio virus, not enough to make you sick, but just enough for the immune army to make polio antibodies, which are then in place to protect you in the future. In the same way, if you're allergic to pollen, when you breathe it in, your body starts to produce antibodies to pollen.

The most familiar symptoms of an allergy include hayfever, a stuffy and running nose, itchy eyes and skin, asthma, headaches, bloating, water retention and facial puffiness. These are signs that your body is trying to get rid of something it doesn't like. Most allergic responses are inflammatory and can bring on pain, swelling and stiffness in the joints and muscles.

Classic food allergies involve the production of an antibody, called immunoglobulin E (IgE), tailored to fit the offending food. IgE-based allergies produce immediate symptoms – such as a rash when eating seafood – and are thus quite easy to detect. However, many allergies involve immunoglobulin G (IgG) reactions. When you have too many IgG reactions occurring in your body, symptoms develop. So your allergic reactions may occur only if you eat a lot of an offending food, or a group of offending foods together. Symptoms are therefore often delayed or hidden and thus harder to detect.

Allergies to food are increasingly common. The most common offenders are dairy products and grains, particularly wheat. However, many other foods cause reactions in some people. But why do some become allergic when others don't?

HAVE YOU GOT LEAKY GUT SYNDROME?

An obvious place to start in unravelling the true cause of allergies is the digestive tract. After all, the lining of the gut is the first point of contact between foods and the immune system. Did you know that the intestinal lining alone is estimated to contain more immune cells and produce more antibodies than any other organ in the body? It's hardly surprising then, that the intestinal lining and its immune system is an absolutely critical defence against food allergens and infections.

In Chapter 8 I explained how the gut can become more leaky (intestinal permeability), allowing incompletely digested food and toxic matter to gain entry into the bloodstream. Research shows that people with food allergies do tend to have leaky gut walls.[60]

IS YOUR IMMUNE SYSTEM WEAKENED?

Another possible reason is that your immune army may be malnourished and hence will over-react to harmless substances. Allergies are therefore much more likely to develop in people who have a weakened immune system, perhaps partly

Food	Per cent of symptomatic patients affected by food		
*Corn	56	Beef	32
**Wheat	54	Coffee	32
Bacon/Pork	39	Malt	27
Oranges	39	Cheese	24
Milk	37	Grapefruit	24
Oats	37	Tomato	22
Rye	34	Peanuts	20
Eggs	32	Sugar (cane)	20

* Corn is the most common in the US   ** Wheat is the most common in the UK

Data from: L G Darlington, 'Dietary therapy for arthritis', *Rheumatic Diseases Clinics of North America*, vol 17(2) (1991), pp. 273–85

Figure 13 – Foods most likely to cause allergy

due to chronic inflammation or poor digestion. The likely allergens are foods eaten frequently, especially those that are potentially irritable to the digestive system (see Figure 13).

As far as arthritis is concerned, the most common suspects are grains and dairy products, followed by pork, beef and eggs. Some people also get relief by avoiding citrus foods and the nightshade family (which includes tomatoes, potatoes, peppers, aubergines and tobacco).

OUR DEADLY BREAD

Although the average person eats between 100g and 200g of wheat every day, in the form of bread, cakes, pasta and cereal, it contains a gastrointestinal irritant called gluten, and is Britain's number-one allergen. Other grains, like rye, barley and oats, also contain gluten. These cause allergic reactions in some people, as does corn (maize). However, rice, buckwheat, millet and quinoa are unlikely to cause allergic reactions.

According to Dr Hicklin, a consultant rheumatologist, grains are the most common allergen in rheumatoid arthritis.[61] He put 22 patients on to a diet excluding likely allergy-provoking foods. No fewer than 20 noted improvements in their symptoms. When tested with different foods, 19 reported that specific foods made them worse, most commonly grains.

According to Dr Nadya Coates, a specialist in grain allergy at the Springhill Foundation in Oxfordshire, gluten has a structure that is alien to the body's metabolism. It sticks to anything and encapsulates smaller molecules, such as sugar, cholesterol, fats or minerals, which are then transported into the blood without being properly digested. Gluten, she

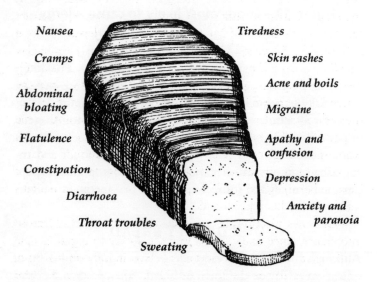

Figure 14 – Symptoms associated with wheat and gluten sensitivity

believes, is the major obstacle in all digestive processes, with wheat gluten being the most toxic of all. Gluten is, unquestionably, an intestinal irritant. In highly sensitive people the lining of the small intestine, which consists of small protrusions called villi, becomes flattened. This is known as coeliac disease and leads to malabsorption, diarrhoea and loss of weight. One study, published in the *Lancet* medical journal, found that almost half of people with rheumatoid arthritis showed gluten sensitivity whereas a quarter of those investigated also had damaged villi.[62] If you have any of the symptoms highlighted in Figure 14, as well as joint pain or stiffness, a trial period off wheat, and possibly off all glutinous grains, is strongly recommended.

MILK ALLERGY

An allergy or intolerance to milk is very common in rheumatoid arthritis sufferers. Consider the case, reported by Dr Panush, Professor of Medicine at the New Jersey Medical School, of a 52-year-old woman who went on a three-day water fast, followed by a hypoallergenic (low allergy-provoking) diet, excluding dairy produce.[63] Within 24 hours of starting the water fast there was noticeable symptomatic relief. She was then given capsules of foods to test. There were no noticeable responses to 52 placebos. Yet on the four separate occasions when she was given milk she reacted every time with a flare-up of symptoms and a raised blood ESR (a measure of inflammation). Many similar reports of dairy allergy in arthritis sufferers have been published.[64]

Sometimes, reactions to dairy products are a result of lactose intolerance, since many adults lose the ability to digest lactose (milk sugar). The usual symptoms are bloating, abdominal pain, wind and diarrhoea, which subside if lactase is taken (the enzyme that breaks down lactose). Probably equally common is an allergy or intolerance to the proteins in dairy produce. For reasons not yet completely understood, the most common symptoms are a blocked nose and excessive mucus production, respiratory problems such as asthma, and gastrointestinal problems. Such intolerances are more likely to occur in people who consume dairy products regularly, in large quantities. Some people who are intolerant of milk can tolerate goat's or sheep's milk better. Butter, which contains virtually no protein, is less likely to cause a reaction.

ONE PERSON'S MEAT IS ANOTHER'S POISON

Other animal proteins, particularly pork, beef and eggs, have also been noted to produce a worsening of arthritic symptoms in susceptible people.[65] Both vegetarian diets that include eggs and dairy products[66] and vegan diets, which exclude all meat, eggs and dairy produce,[67] have produced positive results. One study followed 27 patients who started with a four-week stay at a health farm, where they were placed on a vegan, gluten-free diet which they followed for three and a half months, then gradually moved to a vegetarian diet, including some dairy products and eggs.[68] Participants had remarkable improvements during the initial four weeks and were still showing benefit one year later.

Some arthritis sufferers seem to benefit from the exclusion of foods in the nightshade family (*Solanaceae*), which includes tomatoes, potatoes, aubergine, peppers and tobacco. This regime was made popular by Childers, a horticulturist, who found that this simple exclusion cured his arthritis.[69] Although unproven, these foods do contain solanum alkaloids, which could theoretically inhibit normal collagen repair or promote inflammation. Other suspect foods include peanuts, oranges, grapefruit, malt and coffee.

Coffee also appears to cause inflammation in the body, as shown by the presence of what are known as key inflammatory markers in the blood. A study involving over 3,000 people in

Greece found that those consuming 200ml (7fl oz) of coffee – that's two cups – had between 28 and 30 per cent higher levels of each of these kinds of inflammatory marker compared to non-coffee consumers.[70] Inflammation is now recognised as the basis for many chronic degenerative diseases, including arthritis, so it makes sense to reduce unnecessary exposure to inflammatory agents, particularly when they are also slowing down the liver. I use a simple pin-prick blood test of the liver's detoxification potential, measuring the level of two enzymes – AST and ALT – that indicate how well your liver is detoxing (see page 90).

IDENTIFYING ALLERGIES

Not everyone who has arthritis is allergic or sensitive to certain foods. So how do you know if you are? If you experience three or more of the following symptoms, as well as joint or muscle aches, there is a good chance that you might be allergic:

- hayfever
- a stuffy and running nose
- itchy eyes
- itchy skin
- asthma or difficulty breathing
- headaches
- bloating
- water retention
- facial puffiness
- discoloration around the eyes

If you eat any of the following foods most days and would find them difficult to give up, it's worth testing to see if you're allergic to them:

- wheat (bread, biscuits, cereals, pasta)
- dairy produce (milk, cheese, yogurt)

- meat
- alcohol (especially beer and wine)
- coffee
- chocolate
- peanuts
- eggs
- citrus fruit

PINPOINTING THE ALLERGEN

There are two ways to find out what you are allergic to. The first you could think of as educated 'trial and error'. You need to avoid suspect foods for 14 days and note what happens by taking the pulse test, explained below. Avoid all the substances you suspect may be causing a reaction strictly for 14 days, whether they are on the above list or not. Do check the contents of the foods you eat carefully to see whether they contain any of the above. It is best to stock up on your allergen-free foods before starting.

Wheat

If you are avoiding wheat, stay off all bread, cakes, biscuits, pasta, sauces, cereals, and so on. Alternatives are oatcakes, rice cakes, genuine 100 per cent rye bread such as pumpernickel or volkornbrot, rye crispbread, sauces made with cornflour, corn- or oat-based cereals, and pastry made with corn and almond meal instead of wheat.

Grains

If you are avoiding all grains, stay off anything containing wheat, rye, oats, barley or spelt (an ancient wheat strain). You can eat rice, millet, buckwheat, corn or quinoa. When you reintroduce foods, start with oats, then barley, spelt, rye and lastly wheat.

Milk

If you are avoiding milk, stay off all milk, cheese, yogurt, butter, chocolate and foods containing milk produce. Good alternatives are soya milk, or nut cream (made by blending nuts with water – cashew nuts are particularly good). Drink herb teas that do not require milk. And have more beans, lentils and tofu, if cheese is normally a major source of your protein.

Yeast

If you are avoiding yeast, stay off all breads (unless they are yeast-free), yeast spreads, beer and wine. Be very careful to check the label, especially on baked products.

The pulse test

Most people are free of symptoms within 14 days of avoiding an allergy-provoking food. And most will react within 48 hours on reintroducing the food, although some may have a reaction delayed by up to ten days. Delayed reactions are much harder to test. For some, symptoms improve considerably when they leave out offending foods. For others, noticeable changes are slight. One simple way to help identify possible suspects is the pulse test. The pulse test requires you to avoid all suspect foods for 14 days, then reintroduce them one by one, with a 48-hour gap between each item to be tested.

1   Take your resting pulse, sitting down, before you eat the food, then take it again after 10 minutes, 30 minutes and 60 minutes.
2   Mark all this down on a chart like the one overleaf. If you have a marked increase in pulse rate of more than 10 points, or have any symptoms of ill health

continued

---

within 24 hours including immediate weight gain, bloating, fatigue, headaches or joint aches, for example, avoid the food and wait 24 hours before testing the next food.

Suspect food	Pulse Before	Pulse and Symptoms		
		10 mins	30 mins	60 mins
Egg	_____	_____	_____	_____
Wheat	_____	_____	_____	_____
Milk	_____	_____	_____	_____
Yeast	_____	_____	_____	_____
_____	_____	_____	_____	_____
	_____	_____	_____	_____

Although day-to-day changes in symptoms are hard to pin down to specific causes, avoiding suspect foods for 14 days often lessens symptoms, which then increase significantly when the foods are reintroduced. So you'll be able to pinpoint which foods or drinks make you worse. It is very important to observe symptoms accurately because you may have preconceived ideas about what you do or don't react to, perhaps because of what somebody has told you, or because you dread being allergic to certain foods that you're addicted to.

IGG ALLERGY TESTING – THE GOLD STANDARD

Because the body sometimes delays its allergic reaction to a food, avoidance/reintroduction tests don't always pick the allergy up. This happens because you may not suspect the food, and so don't test it. Or you may suspect only one food, yet be allergic to a range of them, so you'll continue to have a background of allergic reactions.

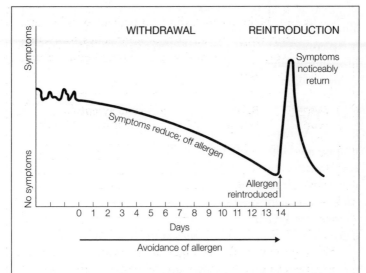

Figure 15 – The avoidance/reintroduction test for allergies

If you avoid a food you are allergic to, you may notice an improvement in how you feel within 14 days. If you then reintroduce the food you may notice a return of symptoms.

Note If you have ever had a severe or life-threatening allergic reaction, I recommend you to do this avoidance/reintroduction test *only* under the supervision of a suitably qualified practitioner.

The best and truly accurate way to find out what you are allergic to is to have what's called a Quantitative IgG ELISA test. This is the gold standard of allergy testing. 'Quantitative' means the test shows not only whether you are allergic, but also how strong your allergic reaction is. Many of us live quite healthily with minor allergies. But stronger allergies can create all kinds of problems, including weight gain. 'ELISA' is the technology used. You don't need to know all the details but it is considered to be the most accurate system. If it's done properly it is at least 93 per cent reproducible. It's used by almost all the best allergy laboratories in the world.

To convey why it's so good, I need to explain a bit about the human immune system.

Your immune system can produce tailor-made weapons that latch onto specific substances to help escort them out of your body. They are like bouncers on the lookout for trouble-makers. As explained on pages 97–8, the bouncers are called immunoglobulins, or Ig for short. There are different types. The real heavies are called IgE, although most allergies involve IgG reactions. IgE reactions tend to be more immediate and severe, such as a violent reaction to peanuts. However, most 'hidden' allergies are IgG-based. In an ideal world you test for both, but I normally start by testing a person for IgG sensitivity to food.

How the testing is done

All that's needed for testing is a pinprick of blood, which is absorbed into a tiny tube and sent to a laboratory. The lab then sends back an accurate readout of exactly what you are aller-gic to. Your body doesn't lie. You either have IgG 'bouncers' tagged for wheat (for example) or you don't. Your diluted blood is introduced to a panel of liquid food 'testers' and, if you've got IgG for that food, a reaction takes place.

There are a number of laboratories who do IgG testing, and one that offers a handy test kit that you can use at home. YorkTest has devised a clever procedure that involves a painless pinprick device and an absorbent material that you place against the pinprick. This material is then sent to the laboratory for testing (see Resources, page 348).

Can you eat those foods again?

The good news about IgG-based allergies is that if you avoid the offending food strictly for three to six months, the body forgets that it is allergic to it. The reason is that there will no longer be any IgG antibodies in your system to that food. So, provided you've removed the underlying cause of the allergy, such as intestinal permeability (leaky gut), and don't overeat that food, there's a good chance that you won't react to it any more. This doesn't hold for IgE-based reactions, however.

To give you an example, I have an IgE allergy to milk. I react within 15 minutes. Even if I avoid dairy products for a year, I still react if I consume one. I used to have an IgG allergy to wheat. I avoided it for three months and now I no longer react. In my case, joint aches weren't the problem: it was migraine headaches. I had them every other week from the age of six to 20, until I discovered that wheat and milk were triggering them.

SUMMARY

If you suspect you are allergic to something in your diet:

- **Test yourself for allergies** with an IgG test or work with your nutritional therapist to investigate any possible allergies or sensitivities. Or …
- **Avoid the suspected foods** for at least 14 days and see if you notice any difference. Do the pulse test when you reintroduce them, one by one (take your pulse before, and 10, 30 and 60 minutes after eating the food again, and make a note of any differences). Observe any changes in your symptoms when you have reintroduced the foods.

For more information about why allergies develop and how to prevent or reverse them, read my book *Hidden Food Allergies* with Dr James Braly (see Recommended Reading, page 343).

CHAPTER 10

UP YOUR ANTIOXIDANTS – THE FREE-RADICAL FIGHTERS

Antioxidant nutrients help reduce inflammation, so if you're an arthritis sufferer or experiencing a lot of pain, eat plenty of fruit (especially berries) and vegetables, or consider supplementing an antioxidant formula. A 2005 UK study involving 25,000 people showed that a low intake of the vitamin antioxidants found in fruit and vegetables significantly increased the risk of arthritis.[71]

Most people are aware that they should be eating at least five portions of fruits and vegetables daily. The World Health Organization takes this one step further and recommends eight to ten servings daily, particularly in relation to cancer prevention. However, a UK government survey revealed that the average adult eats only 2.8 portions daily, and that among 19–24 year olds, only 4 per cent of females and 0 per cent of males achieved this target.

The increased risk of arthritis mentioned above is because one of the major causes of cell damage and inflammation is a process called oxidative stress (or oxidation), caused by too many molecules in the body known as 'free radicals'. A free radical is an atom or group of atoms with an uneven electrical

charge. To complete itself, it steals a charged particle (an elec-
tron) from a neighbouring cell, which can set up a chain reaction producing more free radicals, damaging more cells and
causing them to 'misbehave'. Everyday functions such as
breathing (turning oxygen into carbon dioxide), digestion and
physical activity produce these free radicals, as does exposure
to polluted air, fried or over-cooked food and oxidising radiation from the sun. In fact, in a year our bodies produce almost
a bucketful of such dangerous free radicals, which all have to
be disarmed. So we have developed ways of dealing with these
by-products of using oxygen, through anti-oxidation.

OXIDATION CAUSES DISEASE AND AGEING

A common example of oxidation is when rust attacks metal.
As the rust eats away at the metal, the metal starts to weaken
and decay until it can no longer work. This is what happens to
your body when free radicals attack it. Organs, cells and body
tissues can be weakened by oxidation. This process is what can
lead to diseases such as arthritis, cancer, heart disease and senile
dementia. Eating foods rich in antioxidants neutralises free
radicals and therefore not only helps protect you from life-
threatening disease, but is also thought to slow down the ageing process itself.

Antioxidant nutrients play an important role in inflammation. Antioxidants, like vitamins C and E, protect our cells
from free radical attack and reduce inflammation. Both have
been shown to increase lifespan.[72] Nuts and seeds in their natural state contain vitamin E to protect their essential oils from
oxidation (or rancidity). Yet some oil manufacturers remove
vitamin E and sell us vegetable oil so highly processed that it is
left with little goodness.

According to Dr Richard Cutler, Director of the US
Government Anti-aging Research Department, 'the amount
of antioxidants that you maintain in your body is directly

proportional to how long you will live'. Living in a polluted area, smoking or regularly eating barbecued or deep-fried foods can all create an increased need for antioxidants.

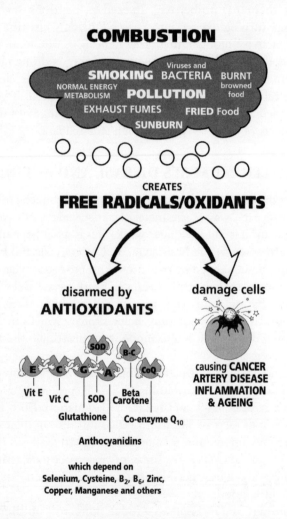

Figure 16 – Antioxidant nutrients and sources of free oxidising radicals

Enzymes in the fight against free radicals

We also have enzymes in our bodies that are designed to disarm free radicals. One of these, SOD (superoxidedismutase), has been the subject of a great deal of arthritis research, which has led to the sale of SOD tablets in health-food stores. Yet there is little evidence that SOD in tablet form can survive the perils of digestion and remain intact to protect us from the damaging effect of free radicals. One type of SOD depends on manganese, deficiency of which results in cartilage problems in joints. Another type of SOD depends on a careful balance of copper and zinc, and yet another type depends on iron. An excess or deficiency of any of these three minerals has also been shown to be associated with worsening symptoms of arthritis. Let me explain why.

IRON – DO WE REALLY NEED EXTRA?

Nowadays, many supplements, as well as drinks, bread and breakfast cereals, sell themselves on their added 'iron'. But do we really need that much? Iron is concentrated in our blood, and is found in every cell in our bodies. Its main role is to combine with protein and copper to make red blood cells, which transport oxygen to each cell. Iron is also needed for the antioxidant enzyme catalase to work. For this reason, having sufficient iron is especially important if you're suffering from an inflammatory disease like arthritis.

Although iron is found in many vegetarian foods, such as beans, lentils, wholegrains, wheatgerm, apricots and eggs, the iron in meat is much more easily absorbed by the body. Eating vitamin C-rich foods with vegetarian sources of iron increases the amount of iron absorbed. So, for example, scrambled eggs on wholegrain toast with a glass of orange juice would deliver significant amounts of iron.

Finding balance

Iron is one of the few minerals doctors are keen to prescribe, especially for pregnant women. Although it is true that around one in ten people are iron-deficient, too much iron can also be bad and can induce zinc deficiency. Once again, it's all a question of balance. In practical terms, it is not wise to supplement more than 15mg of iron unless a test has been run to determine that a person is definitely iron-deficient, and extra zinc is given as well.

Iron levels in the joints and synovial fluid of arthritis sufferers, particularly rheumatoid arthritis, are usually considerably higher than in people without arthritis.[73] Levels in the blood are usually low, possibly indicating that ongoing inflammation uses up iron reserves. This is thought to indicate that iron (as part of the antioxidant army fighting against inflammation and joint damage) is needed in larger amounts. In most cases, when a bout of inflammation is over, synovial iron levels decrease and blood levels increase.

When is it appropriate to supplement?

For some people, supplementation of substantial levels of iron may be unwise. One woman, diagnosed as iron-deficient, supplemented her diet, and within three days her arthritis symptoms were much worse. Once off the iron supplements, she got better. Another patient, diagnosed as iron-deficient, had initial relief of iron-deficiency symptoms after taking iron supplements, but then went on to develop severe rheumatoid arthritis within two weeks. On investigation, her hands and feet showed long-term erosive changes consistent with rheumatoid arthritis, but, until she took the iron, she had had no symptoms and no pain.[74]

There are two possible explanations for these unusual stories. The first is that iron is needed for the body's normal inflammatory responses, probably as part of catalase, the antioxidant enzyme. In cases of iron deficiency the body is unable to respond in the normal way (hence the absence of pain), although the joint degeneration clearly takes place. Once the iron deficiency is corrected, inflammation starts. There may be an element of truth in this theory, but one would not expect excessive inflammation.

The other possible, and perhaps more plausible, explanation is this. Free radicals are dangerous oxides that damage joint tissue. In order to disarm the free radical it must first be acted on by the enzyme catalase, which is dependent on iron. This enzyme does not actually disarm the free radical. It is still dangerous, but it is now in a form in which it can be disarmed by other antioxidants.

If someone in an active stage of inflammation was given extra iron, this could, in fact, increase free radical activity.[75] Presumably, if they were given a sufficient amount of other antioxidants this would minimise this possibility. The point is that taking in too much iron can encourage oxidation and inflammation.

At this point I can conclude that there are potential dangers in over-prescribing iron, and potential benefits in prescribing it for some arthritic patients. It may be far safer to take an all-round multimineral supplement containing zinc, manganese, selenium and small amounts of iron and copper, to maintain the right balance of these essential trace elements.

THE ZINC LINK

Zinc, like iron, is part of the antioxidant enzyme SOD, and is involved in inflammation. Like iron, high levels tend to be found in the synovial fluid of people with arthritis,[76] whereas other body indicators show low levels. The assumption here is that zinc is used up at a faster rate when there is an ongoing active inflammatory disease such as arthritis. Zinc is vital for over 200 of the body's known enzymes, especially in relation to healthy immune function, growth, repair and protein utilisation. So, theoretically, it is necessary to have adequate zinc for cartilage repair, proper immune and inflammatory responses, and warding off viruses and other infections.

It is not only in theory that zinc is good for arthritis; it has proven beneficial in a research trial published in the *Lancet*.[77] Here, 24 patients with chronic rheumatoid arthritis were given 220mg of zinc or an identical dummy pill three times a day for 12 weeks. At the end of 12 weeks all the patients were given zinc. During the first 12-week period those who took zinc had less joint swelling and less morning stiffness, could walk further and generally felt better than those on the dummy pills. When those previously taking the dummy pills started taking zinc they also improved.

This trial was repeated with a group of psoriatic arthritis sufferers, again with positive results.[78] (Psoriatic arthritis affects around 10–30 per cent of people suffering from the chronic skin condition psoriasis.) The most significant effects, which included less joint pain and less morning stiffness, were seen after five weeks on zinc. These improvements were accompanied by a reduction in serum immunoglobulins (antibodies in the blood), which suggested that these patients had a less 'reactive' immune system after taking zinc supplements.

However, a third trial, using the same amount of zinc in severe long-standing rheumatoid arthritis sufferers, found improvement in only six out of 22 patients.[79] This may have been because a single nutrient cannot usually act in isolation. A combination of factors is normally required.

Zinc is also vital for proper digestion. Protein cannot be digested without the combination of hydrochloric acid in the stomach and protein-digesting enzymes. The production of both these substances depends on zinc. So zinc deficiency could lead to poor protein digestion, paving the way for gut reactions to undigested proteins, possibly precipitating food allergies that encourage joint inflammation. There is evidence that arthritis sufferers may produce insufficient amounts of hydrochloric acid.[80]

Where can we find natural sources?

Zinc is not only vital for us, it's vital for plants too. That's why nuts, seeds and the germ of grains, such as wheat or oats, are all good sources of zinc. Animal produce also supplies zinc, as it is required for the development of all new cells. The richest known source of zinc is oysters. Refined food has virtually no zinc and most vegetables and fruit contain little, unless you eat the seeds. Sesame and sunflower seeds are good sources of zinc because they also contain calcium, magnesium, selenium and vitamin E. I have a spoonful of ground-up seeds on my cereal or in a salad every day.

Zinc is probably the most commonly lacking mineral in the UK. Deficiency signs include poor taste or sense of smell, frequent infections, stretch marks, acne or greasy skin, pale skin, tendency to depression, low fertility and loss of appetite. The average intake of zinc is around 8mg a day, which falls a long way short of the World Health Organization's recommended intake of 15mg a day. Apart from not getting enough from the diet, there are also instances when the body's need for zinc is increased, such as at times of stress, infections, PMS, hormonal imbalances, using the contraceptive pill, frequent alcohol consumption, and blood sugar problems (for example, in diabetes). Someone with ongoing inflammation may need up to 25mg a day. With the right kind of diet, you can guarantee an intake of 10–15mg a day, leaving a possible deficit of up to 15mg, which is why I recommend supplementing 10–15mg of zinc every day, as well as eating a zinc-rich diet.

CAN COPPER CAUSE ARTHRITIS?

Copper is an essential mineral for the body. It is involved in the antioxidant enzyme SOD and reduces inflammation in the joints. It also helps to make red blood cells and the insulating layer around nerves. However, copper can also be toxic if you get too much, as the story of a patient of mine illustrates.

Case Study: Mrs M

Mrs M's osteoarthritis had been getting continually worse over the previous five years. No conventional treatment had helped ease the pain in her joints and even changing her diet and taking vitamin supplements had done little for her. I asked her if anything improved her condition. She said that she only felt better when she stayed at a friend's cottage in the country. She had once tried a copper bracelet, but that had made her worse. A hair mineral analysis revealed that she had copper levels three times higher than normal. The most common source of excess copper is copper water pipes. If the plumbing is new, or the water is soft, significant amounts of copper leach into water. Mrs M drank plenty of water from the tap, except when she stayed at her friend's cottage where the water came from a spring. Could it be that she was being poisoned by too much copper in her water?

The problem with excess copper is that it competes with zinc. Both are needed to fight inflammation. However, too much copper and not enough zinc could make inflammation worse, not better. Drinking large quantities of water passing through copper pipes can give you more than enough, as explained above, especially if the copper plumbing is new, which means the pipes and joints have yet to be calcified.

On average, we need at least ten times as much zinc as copper. If your intake of copper comes from whole foods (including nuts, seeds, lentils, beans and fruits), this is fine, because they also contain zinc. However, if your diet does not include such foods, and you drink unfiltered water that passes through copper pipes, you could accumulate too much. Taking the birth control pill also increases the retention of copper.

THE BENEFITS OF COPPER

Copper levels in the blood and joints of people with arthritis are often very high. One study found three times as much copper in the synovial fluid of rheumatoid arthritis sufferers.[81] But, rather than being a sign of toxicity, these high copper levels are thought to occur precisely because the body is fighting inflammation. Zinc and iron levels are also often raised. When arthritis sufferers go into remission, copper levels fall. However, during active arthritis, stores of copper in the liver fall. This suggests that the requirement for copper is greater in an arthritis sufferer. Many studies have also shown greater benefit from supplementing copper salicylate, rather than just salicylic acid (aspirin), suggesting again that copper has an important anti-inflammatory effect.

This may explain why some people benefit from copper bracelets. The benefit of copper bracelets was put to the test in one study where 240 arthritic patients were given either a copper bracelet or a placebo bracelet to wear for a month.[82] After a month, those with the copper bracelet were given a placebo bracelet and vice versa. It was found that those who noted a difference in their condition between month one and month two, had significantly improved when wearing the copper bracelet. Those who had previously worn a copper bracelet, and then wore the placebo bracelet, got worse.

So, copper can help or hinder you, depending on your current copper status. I recommend a hair-mineral analysis or an equivalent test for any arthritis sufferer. Such a test also gives useful information about other minerals. See my website (www.patrickholford.com) to locate a nutritional therapist in your area who can carry out these tests.

BOOST YOUR SELENIUM INTAKE

Going back to antioxidant enzymes, there is another that is closely related to SOD called GP (glutathione peroxidase), which depends on the mineral selenium. Increase the dietary intake of selenium by a factor of ten and you will double the activity of GP.[83]

WHY IS SELENIUM VITAL?

Forty years ago, selenium was known only as a toxic mineral. Now it is recognised as one of the most essential trace elements for the human body. In both animals and man, high selenium intake is associated with low risk of cancer. A deficiency increases the risk of cancer, heart disease and arthritis. US and UK governments are currently sponsoring research to find out just how much selenium we need to prevent these major diseases.

Many crops are grown in soils with a low selenium content and this results in a correspondingly low level of selenium in the produce. Refining foods also lowers selenium content.

A number of studies have found low levels of selenium in arthritic patients.[84] One study checked 26 girls with juvenile arthritis; another checked adults with rheumatoid arthritis. Levels tended to be lowest in people with the most severe symptoms. Levels of the selenium-dependent enzyme GP were also low.

Selenium supplementation has recently been shown to be effective in the treatment of rheumatoid arthritis.[85] Dr Peretz, at the Department of Rheumatology at Brugmann Hospital in Brussels, gave eight patients 200mcg of selenium per day, and compared them with seven patients given placebo supplements. According to Dr Peretz, 'pain and joint involvement [stiffness] were reduced in most (six out of eight) patients treated with selenium while the placebo group showed no significant modification'. In his opinion, selenium probably works by stimulating GP enzyme activity, which detoxifies the free radicals that are generated in large amounts in inflammatory rheumatic diseases.

In a German study of people with rheumatoid arthritis, those given selenium and fish oils over three months had less tender or swollen joints and less morning stiffness than those just given fish oils. Those on the selenium also needed less cortisone and NSAID medication, and laboratory tests showed that they had less inflammation.[86]

Where can we find natural sources?

The best food sources of selenium are seafood, seaweed and sesame seeds.

VITAMINS C AND E

Vitamin C has been found to be low in rheumatoid arthritis sufferers,[87] possibly because, as a free radical scavenger, vitamin C sacrifices itself in the process of fighting free radicals. (And inflammation in the areas affected by rheumatoid arthritis increases free radical activity.)

But vitamin C is not only an antioxidant. It is also necessary for cartilage and bone formation. Collagen cannot be synthesised without vitamin C; deficiency causes severe signs of osteoarthritis in guinea pigs, who, like us, are not able to synthesise their own vitamin C.[88] Whereas guinea pigs given sufficient amounts of vitamin C do not develop osteoarthritis. Both vitamins C and E help to control the synthesis of proteoglycans, which helps the formation of cartilage.

As long ago as 1964, vitamin C was found to relieve back pain, possibly by helping to preserve disc integrity.[89] More recently there have been reports of positive results using 'Ester-C', a vitamin C product that contains the metabolites produced from vitamin C. (Metabolites are substances produced by chemical reactions in your body, i.e. the intermediate steps of metabolism.) There is some evidence that these metabolites may be much more effective than vitamin C itself. Dr Edwin Goertz, a Canadian physician, has used Ester-C with 300 patients, with good results. According to him, 'At least 5 per cent have reported good results in their symptoms using Ester-C either as a primary treatment or as an adjunctive therapy.'[90]

Since vitamin C is a water-soluble antioxidant and vitamin E is a fat-soluble antioxidant, protecting fatty layers of cells, the combination of these two nutrients may well help reduce inflammation and speed up healing of joints. The recommended intake of vitamin E is up to 500iu per day, whereas the recommended intake of vitamin C is 3–10g per day.

Where can we find natural sources?

The best food sources of vitamin C are peppers, broccoli, berries, kiwi fruit and citrus fruit such as oranges and lemons.

THE VALUE OF VITAMIN E

Vitamin E is a valuable ally in the fight against inflammation because of its antioxidant and membrane-stabilising properties. There is little question that a deficiency increases free radical activity within joints,[91] and that supplementing vitamin E reduces this potential cause of inflammation.[92] In animals, a lack of vitamin E has been shown to cause arthritis, which can be reversed by ensuring optimal intakes of this vital antioxidant.[93] The first study to be published, from St Bartholomew's Hospital in London, found that in people with rheumatoid arthritis vitamin E had a significant painkilling effect, although clinical measurements of their inflammation showed little change after the three-month trial.[94] The researchers believed that the painkilling effect could be due to vitamin E's ability to quench nitric oxide radicals that are involved in the transmission of pain.

According to research in the US, many arthritis sufferers may not get anywhere near enough vitamin E to limit inflammation.[95] In a diet survey, 20 out of 24 rheumatoid arthritis sufferers, and 11 out of 12 osteoarthritis sufferers, consumed less than half the RDA for vitamin E. Intakes of vitamin E in the order of 500iu per day have been shown to ease arthritis.

Where can we find natural sources?

The best food sources of vitamin E are unrefined corn oils, sunflower seeds, sesame seeds and wheatgerm.

QUERCETIN

Many of the natural painkillers we discussed in Chapter 5 are also potent antioxidants. Quercetin is a good example.

A trial in which people with rheumatoid arthritis were treated with a vegan diet high in antioxidants including quercetin found they had decreased joint stiffness and pain as well as an improvement in self-reported health.[96]

How much to take

Take between 300mg and 600mg per day, between meals.

OTHER ANTIOXIDANTS

There are literally hundreds of antioxidants in foods. Although vitamins A, C and E, and selenium, have been most extensively investigated, other key antioxidants include glutathione (found in white meat, seafood, lentils, beans, nuts and seeds), co-enzyme Q_{10} (found in sardines, mackerel and soya oil) and anthocyanidins (found in red-blue foods such as berries and beetroot). These work together in disarming free radicals and reducing the risk of inflammation. For example, vitamin E, once it has neutralised free radicals, can be recycled by vitamin C. Vitamin C can be recycled by glutathione and glutathione can, in turn, be recycled by anthocyanidins.

What you want is a combination of the most powerful antioxidants: vitamins C and E, glutathione or N-acetyl-cysteine, lipoic acid and co-enzyme Q_{10}. If you are in constant pain, it could be well worth taking extra amounts of these in supplement form for a while – but ideally, in addition to eating a diet rich in fruit and vegetables, and increasing your intake of fish, seeds, nuts, eggs, onions and garlic.

As you saw earlier, many of the plant extracts that we recommend for their anti-inflammatory effects also have powerful antioxidant effects – one of the most exciting being those from olives, called hydroxytyrosol (explained in Chapter 5).

ARE YOU GETTING ENOUGH ANTIOXIDANTS?

Researchers have devised a measure of the antioxidant levels in foods called ORAC ('oxygen radical absorbency capacity' for the technically minded). The oldest living people are thought to consume at least 6,000 ORACs a day.

The chart opposite shows ORAC ratings of 20 different foods that you can easily incorporate into your diet. Each serving contains about 2,000 units. Just pick three of these daily to hit your anti-ageing score of 6,000. The complete chart is available on my website at www.patrickholford.com/ORAC.

20 top foods to add ten years to your life

1 ⅓ tsp cinnamon, ground

2 ½ tsp oregano, dried

3 ½ tsp turmeric, ground

4 1 heaped tsp mustard

5 ⅕ cup blueberries

6 Half a pear, grapefruit or plum

7 ½ cup blackcurrants or berries such as raspberries, strawberries

8 ½ cup cherries or a shot of CherryActive concentrate (see box, page 126)

9 An orange or apple

10 4 pieces of dark chocolate (70% cocoa solids)

11 7 walnut halves

12 8 pecan halves

13 ¼ cup pistachio nuts

14 ½ cup cooked lentils

15 1 cup cooked kidney beans

16 ⅓ medium avocado

17 ½ cup of red cabbage

18 2 cups of broccoli

19 1 medium globe artichoke or 8 spears of asparagus

20 medium glass/150ml (¼ pint) red wine

Source: *Oxygen Radical Absorbance Capacity of Selected Foods*, US Department of Agriculture (2007)

Go for flavour and colour

Generally speaking, where you find the most colour and flavour you will also find the highest antioxidant levels. The reds, yellows and oranges of tomatoes and carrots, for example are due to the presence of beta-carotene. Globe artichoke has the highest rating of vegetables, whereas other vegetables, such as carrots, peas and spinach are lower in units, so aim for five to ten servings daily of a range of fruits and vegetables to keep your intake high.

Fruits that have the highest levels are those with the deepest colour, such as blueberries, raspberries and strawberries. These are particularly rich in powerful antioxidants called proanthocyanidins. One cup of blueberries, for example, will provide 9,697 units. You would need to eat 11 bananas to get the same benefit as a cupful of blueberries!

The number of portions needed per day really does depend on your choices, as you can see in the menus below. Both days have five portions selected, but the Day 1 selection is 8,001 less than Day 2.

Our daily choices *do* make a difference!

Day 1 Fruit/vegetable portion	ORAC	Day 2 Fruit/vegetable portion	ORAC
⅛ large cantaloupe melon	315	½ pear	2,617
kiwi fruit	802	½ cup strawberries	2,683
1 medium carrot, raw	406	½ avocado	2,899
cup green peas, frozen	432	1 cup broccoli, raw	1,226
1 cup spinach, raw	455	4 spears asparagus, boiled	986
Total score	**2,410**	**Total score**	**10,411**

Cherries for health

Did you know that it is possible to get an anti-ageing hit of 23 portions of fruit and veg in a single glass of juice? Sounds amazing, but a delicious cherry concentrate delivers just that!

CherryActive is made from tart Montmorency cherries and each 30ml serving has an impressive ORAC (or antioxidant) score of 8,260. To put this in perspective, five servings of fruit and vegetables have an ORAC score of around 1,750 units. The chart below shows a typical day's selection.

Typical five-a-day food portions	ORAC units*
Medium banana (80g**)	650
Watermelon (80g)	113
Fresh tomatoes (80g)	294

continued

Garden peas (80g)	480
Cooked carrots (80g)	253
Total for selected five-a-day	**1,790**
CherryActive Concentrate (30ml) (makes one 280ml glass of cherry juice when diluted with water)	**8,260**

Source: *Oxygen Radical Absorbance Capacity of Selected Foods*, US Department of Agriculture (2007)
**80g is the standard portion measure for the UK government's five-a-day programme

In case you are wondering, you cannot have too many antioxidants in your diet – your body will use what it needs and excrete the rest. However, antioxidants work synergistically, so if taking them in supplement form they should not be taken in isolation, especially in large amounts.

SUMMARY

To increase your antioxidants, follow these top tips:
- **Aim to eat five to ten servings** of fruits, vegetables, nuts and spices daily – and think colour.
- **When preparing meals**, aim to fill at least half your plate with vegetables.
- **Heating destroys antioxidants**, so aim to eat most of your fruits and vegetables raw or lightly cooked.
- **Stock up on frozen berries** and add to yogurt or use to make smoothies or home-made ice-cream.
- **Keep a bowl of fruit** on your desk at work.
- **Snack on fruit and raw nuts** rather than crisps. A handful of nuts with fruit will also help to keep your blood sugar balanced.

CHAPTER 11

BENEFICIAL B VITAMINS

The B vitamins are vital for all-round health. As they are not stored in the body, a daily supply is necessary for energy production, healthy nerves, good skin and a host of other roles, including hormone and prostaglandin production (both important in controlling arthritic diseases). They are also needed to keep your homocysteine at a healthy level; I'll explain all about homocysteine in this chapter. One B vitamin – B_5 – is directly involved in the production of cortisone. Vitamin B_5 is also called pantothenic acid, from the Greek word *pantos* (meaning 'everywhere') because it is found in so many foods. Despite this, many people do not get enough of this essential nutrient, which is also needed to make energy in every single cell. In addition, it helps make acetylcholine, an important chemical in the brain that is thought to be involved in memory.

VITAMIN B_5 (PANTOTHENIC ACID)

As long ago as 1950 it was known that animals severely deficient in pantothenic acid developed osteoarthritis, including osteoporosis, calcification of cartilage and the formation of osteophytes.[97] This led Dr Annand in Dundee to experiment with giving his osteoarthritic patients pantothenic acid.[98] He found that a supplement of 12.5mg each morning and evening produced an improvement in their condition and a drop in their ESR (a measurement of inflammation). The improvement did not appear for seven to ten days. And, stopping the supplements, the symptoms returned.

People with rheumatoid arthritis have been found to be particularly lacking in B$_5$. A study of 66 arthritis patients found their blood levels of pantothenic acid to be very much lower than those without arthritis.[99] This study also found that vegetarians tended to have higher levels than those eating a 'normal' diet. This is not surprising since vegetables are a good source of pantothenic acid.

So, the researchers asked, could pantothenic acid also help rheumatoid arthritis sufferers? They decided to test this theory, by giving 20 patients with low pantothenic acid levels injections of this B vitamin for a month. Within seven days both their symptoms and their blood levels of pantothenic acid had improved. Once the intravenous pantothenic acid was stopped, blood levels again dropped and the symptoms returned.

This study was repeated under more rigorous conditions 17 years later, using oral supplements instead of injections.[100] Eighteen rheumatoid arthritis patients were given either 500mg of pantothenic acid four times a day (as calcium pantothenate) or a placebo. After two months there was a reduction in morning stiffness, severity of pain and disability in those taking the pantothenic acid.

How does pantothenic acid work?

Exactly how pantothenic acid works is still a bit of a mystery. But we do know that it is required for the production of corticosteroids, the body's natural anti-inflammatory agents. And this may explain the improvement in rheumatoid arthritis. However, the formation of osteoarthritis-like joint changes seen in animals with a deficiency suggests a role in joint health, perhaps by affecting calcium balance.

Pantothenic acid is certainly worth trying for any form of arthritis. I know of no trials to date using significant amounts of pantothenic acid that have failed to show a positive response.

How much to take

I recommend 500–1,000mg pantothenic acid each day for any arthritis sufferer for a trial period of two months. Pantothenic acid supplementation may also help gout (a build-up of uric acid in the body), since it helps convert uric acid to urea and ammonia, which can be eliminated from the body.

Where can we find natural sources?

The best food sources of vitamin B_5 are mushrooms, eggs and lentils.

VITAMIN B_3 (NIACINAMIDE)

Another B vitamin that has proved helpful for arthritis sufferers is vitamin B_3, also known as niacin or niacinamide. Niacinamide has been used with good results since 1943. It is interesting to note that today's resistance to nutritional therapy existed more than 40 years ago. In the 1950s Dr William Kaufman, who pioneered this research, wrote to Dr Abram Hoffer:

> 'Ever since 1943 I have tried to call my work on niacinamide
> to the attention of leading rheumatologists, nutritionists and
> gerontologists through conversations with them, by sending
> them copies of my monographs and papers on this subject, and
> by two talks given on the usefulness of niacinamide and other
> vitamins which I gave at the International Gerontological
> Congresses in 1951 and 1954. I think that two factors have
> made it difficult for doctors to accept the concept that

continuous therapy with large doses of niacinamide could cause improvement in joint dysfunction and give other benefits: (a) the advent of cortisone, and (b) the fact that my use of vitamins was such a departure from the recommended daily allowance for vitamins by the National Research Council.'

Dr Hoffer had contacted Dr Kaufman after coincidentally finding that some of his patients whom he was treating with high doses of niacin, either for schizophrenia or for high cholesterol levels, were reporting improvement in their arthritis.[101] He noted six cases of osteo- and rheumatoid arthritis who received either niacin or niacinamide in doses of 1,000–3,000mg per day, four of whom experienced a complete recovery, one of whom was described as 'nearly normal', and the last as much improved.

Case Study: Mrs HC

Here is an excerpt from the case of Mrs HC, who was diagnosed with osteoarthritis at the age of 68 in February 1954:

'Her hands were becoming deformed and showed marked ulnar deviation, well-marked Heberden's nodes on all fingers, and severe pain on movement. In March 1954, she was started on 1g niacin per day in two divided doses. She has continued on this medication until the present report (1959). About three months later (July 1954) I again examined the patient. There was a marked improvement, mentally and physically. She no longer complained of neuritis; her vision became normal and has not failed her since. The ulnar deviation of her hands vanished, as did the Heberden's nodes. These nodes went through an interesting change. In random order they first enlarged somewhat, then receded in size until they became hardly visible. Her hands became normally mobile. The skin regained its previous elasticity and tone.'

Dr William Kaufman devised a simple, objective method for determining joint mobility, and set to work recording the effects of niacinamide therapy, which he gave in doses of 900–4,000mg per day, in divided doses, with or without other vitamins. By 1955 he had recorded the effects of niacinamide on 663 patients.[102] He showed conclusively that, without exception, patients who took adequate amounts of niacinamide on a continuous basis had significant and measurable improvement in joint mobility and function, less stiffness, less joint deformity and lowered ESR levels. These results were seen in rheumatoid and osteoarthritis sufferers and continued as long as the supplementation was continued. Stopping the supplements resulted in worsening of symptoms.

However, it wasn't until 1996 that his method was tested in a proper double-blind study by researchers at the US National Institutes of Health. Their results were equally encouraging and confirmed that those taking vitamin B_3, compared with the control group, had overall improvement, less inflammation, more mobility in their joints and were able to reduce their anti-inflammatory medication.[103] High-dose niacin is also one of the most effective ways to lower high cholesterol levels, and increase the good HDL cholesterol.[104]

HOW MUCH B_3 IS SAFE?

The niacin form of vitamin B_3, which is the most effective for lowering high cholesterol levels, causes a blushing sensation. This usually lasts for up to 30 minutes and is not harmful, although some people find it unpleasant. However, neither niacinamide nor inositol hexanicotinate cause blushing. Although I am aware of no reports of toxicity of niacinamide at the levels used by Dr Kaufman, I would be cautious about supplementing more than 2,000mg per day of any form of B_3 without the guidance and supervision of a doctor or clinical nutritional therapist. This level, however, would appear to be entirely safe.[105] We know an awful lot about adverse effects of high-dose niacin from its use in lowering cholesterol. Some people taking the blushing form report nausea and gastrointestinal upset.

Where can we find natural sources?

The best food sources of vitamin B_3 are turkey, chicken, tuna and mackerel.

VITAMIN B_6 (PYRIDOXINE)

Another vitamin that relieves symptoms of arthritis is vitamin B_6, or pyridoxine. Dr John Ellis, from Mount Pleasant in Texas, found that giving B_6 in doses of 50mg helped to control pain and restore joint mobility to his patients.[106] Vitamin B_6 shrinks the synovial membranes that line the bearing surfaces of the joints. It also helps to regulate the synthesis of anti-inflammatory prostaglandins.

Dr Ellis also found another use for this vitamin – the relief of a nerve disorder called carpal tunnel syndrome. This painful and crippling disease affects the hands and wrists, and is caused by compression of the principal nerve supply for the hand as it passes through a tunnel lined with synovial membrane, between the tendons and ligaments in the wrist. A double-blind controlled study by Ellis and Karl Folkers, a professor at the University of Austin, Texas, proved that B_6 was so effective that, in the authors' words, 'pyridoxine therapy may frequently obviate hand surgery'.[107]

Why, you may ask, when all the evidence is there to support the use of these inexpensive nutrients, are so few doctors paying any attention? Part of the answer is that we do need more clinical trials, but most trials cost in excess of £1million and, unless there's a patentable, profitable drug at the end of it, who's going to pay for this kind of research?

Where can we find natural sources?

The best food sources of vitamin B_6 are Brussels sprouts, bananas, red kidney beans and cauliflower.

FOLIC ACID AND VITAMIN B_{12}

The effectiveness of these two B vitamins was demonstrated in an experiment on 26 people who had been suffering from osteoarthritis of the hands for an average of more than five years and had been taking NSAIDs. The only drug the participants took during the trial was paracetamol, for pain relief when it was needed. Otherwise, the results showed that those taking a combination of vitamin B_{12} and folic acid had less tenderness in their hand joints, and had similar improvement in the ability of their hands to grip objects and had no side effects compared with those on NSAIDs.[108] NSAIDs, on the other hand, do cause side effects and they cost more than B_{12} and folic acid supplements.

Appropriate daily doses would be 200mcg of folic acid and, at least, 10mcg of B_{12}.

Where can we find natural sources?

The best food sources of folic acid are wheatgerm, spinach, broccoli, beans, nuts and seeds. The best food sources of vitamin B_{12} are sardines, oysters and seafood.

HOMOCYSTEINE

In recent years I've been explaining why your homocysteine level is your greatest single health statistic. The level of homocysteine in your blood is a better indicator than your blood pressure, your cholesterol level, or even your weight, of whether you will live a long and healthy life or die young. As high levels of homocysteine are associated with inflammation, finding out your homocysteine level and then reducing it if necessary could make a marked difference to the discomfort of your condition, as I will explain.

Case Study: Valerie

Valerie, aged 73, had suffered from high blood pressure for over 30 years, as well as a touch of arthritis. Her doctor had given her two drugs, Captopril and a junior aspirin every day. They had helped her a bit, but her blood pressure was still high, often as high as 160/80.

She decided to have a homocysteine test. Her homocysteine score was 42.9, putting her in the very high-risk category (as a healthy level is below 6), so she went on my diet and the supplement programme recommended in my book *The H Factor*. After two months she retested and her H score had dropped by 88 per cent to a healthy 5.1. Her blood pressure had also dropped and stabilised at 132/80 and she no longer needed any medication. Her arthritis improved too, causing her much less joint pain and she felt altogether much better in herself.

What is homocysteine?

Homocysteine is a type of protein produced in the body from the amino acid methionine, which is found in normal dietary protein. Homocysteine in itself isn't bad news – your body naturally turns it into one of two beneficial substances. Ideally it should be present in very low quantities in the blood. However, if you don't have the optimal amount of B vitamins and other vital nutrients in your diet, homocysteine can accumulate, increasing your risk of over 50 diseases, including arthritis, heart disease, stroke, certain cancers, diabetes, depression and Alzheimer's disease. This is because the enzymes that turn homocysteine into either glutathione or SAMe, don't work efficiently, so blood homocysteine levels increase (see Figure 17). (Glutathione is the body's most important antioxidant – see Chapter 10; SAMe – S-adenosyl methione – is a very important type of 'intelligent' nutrient for both brain and body, participating in over 40 essential biochemical reactions.) The good news is that, with the right nutrients, this important risk factor can be reversed.

It has also been discovered that the enzyme that converts homocysteine into SAMe (it's called the MTHFR enzyme) doesn't work as well in some people (approximately one in ten) due to an inherited genetic mutation. For these individuals to stay healthy, larger intakes of vitamin B_{12} and folic acid are necessary.

What does homocysteine tell us?

So why does the body make homocysteine and what does a high level tell us? It's all to do with a fundamental process upon which your life depends. It's called methylation, which happens over a billion times a second. Every second there are hundreds of thousands of adjustments made in your body to keep you healthy and alive. For example, when your body is under stress, the body makes more adrenalin to keep you going. When you go to bed, the body releases melatonin to help you sleep. When you've got a cold or flu the body makes more glutathione, which turns your immune cells into cold-busting warriors. It is like one big dance, with biochemicals in your body passing 'methyl groups' (made of one carbon and three hydrogen atoms) from one partner to another.

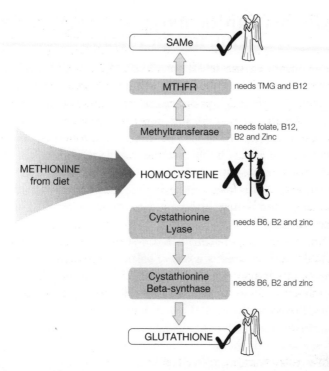

Figure 17 – The homocysteine pathway

We all make homocysteine from eating protein. Normally, it is quickly turned into SAMe or glutathione, two very essential and health-promoting substances in the body. But if you lack enough of certain nutrients such as B_2, B_6, B_{12}, folic acid, zinc, or tri-methyl glycine (TMG), you end up accumulating toxic homocysteine.

It is also thought that methylation plays a critical role in protecting us from certain serious diseases. Methyl groups are added to and subtracted from our DNA. When not enough methylation is going on, our DNA cannot properly repair itself, which puts us at higher risk of cancer and autoimmune diseases such as rheumatoid arthritis or lupus.

RHEUMATOID ARTHRITIS SUFFERERS HAVE HIGH HOMOCYSTEINE

High homocysteine levels are linked to most inflammatory diseases, since they promote arachidonic acid release, an increase in PGE2 (pro-inflammatory prostaglandins, as explained in Chapter 5) and hence inflammation.[109] When the body has lost its ability to methylate properly, which is what having a high homocysteine level is all about, pain and inflammation are just around the corner. Homocysteine levels are frequently found to be higher in rheumatoid arthritis sufferers,[110] and may contribute to their increased risk of heart disease.[111]

Since rheumatoid arthritis is a 'systemic' disease, where the whole body's chemistry is out of balance and many tissues and organs other than the joints are affected, one would suspect that homocysteine plays a leading role in the disease. And it does. Research from the Department of Biochemistry at the University Hospital in Madrid, Spain, examined the H scores of women with rheumatoid arthritis versus those without.[112] There was a massive difference. The average H score for those with rheumatoid arthritis was a sky-high 17.3, compared to 7.6 for those without!

Other research groups have found similar differences, especially among rheumatoid arthritis sufferers with a history of thrombosis,[113] or abnormal clotting of blood. Homocysteine has also been implicated in ankylosing spondylitis, an inflammatory, crippling arthritic disease of the spine.[114]

Homocysteine is thought to damage joints[115] and other tissue directly, as do oxidants produced by the body. Remember, the presence of high homocysteine levels means there's less glutathione available. This incredibly powerful antioxidant minimises the damage wreaked by oxidants. When it's deficient – as with high homocysteine – the oxidants take over, accelerating the destruction of joint tissues. This can speed the development of both rheumatoid arthritis and osteoarthritis. The low SAMe levels that hit when homocysteine is high are also significant here, as SAMe has proven anti-osteoarthritic benefits.

All of this suggests that reducing homocysteine may well help those with arthritis considerably. Yet, disappointingly, very little research has yet been done to test the homocysteine theory of arthritis. An exception occurred in 1994 when forward-thinking researchers from the highly esteemed American College of Nutrition in Clearwater, Florida, gave B_{12} and folate supplements to 26 people who had been suffering from osteoarthritis of the hands for an average of more than five years, and had been taking NSAIDs. The results showed that people with arthritis who took the vitamins in place of the NSAIDs had less tenderness in their hand joints, and similar improvement in their ability to grip objects, compared with those just taking NSAIDs, but none of the notorious side effects seen with the use of these drugs.[116] NSAIDs can cause serious reactions, including premature death from kidney failure, ulcers and bleeding in the digestive tract, and they cost considerably more than B_{12} and folate supplements.

Vitamin B_6, another homocysteine-lowering vitamin, may also help arthritis sufferers. Back in the 1950s, an insightful physician from Mount Pleasant in Texas, Dr John Ellis, found that giving B_6 in higher daily doses of 50mg helped to control pain and restore joint mobility to his arthritic patients.[117] Vitamin B_6 shrinks inflamed membranes that line the weight-bearing surfaces of the joints, perhaps by helping decrease homocysteine and increasing SAMe and glutathione, both proven anti-inflammatory agents. B_6 also helps to regulate production of the prostaglandins, the body's own anti-inflammatory agents. I predict that following a homocysteine-lowering programme will produce even more spectacular results.

DRUGS THAT RAISE HOMOCYSTEINE

A relatively small number of prescribed medical drugs used for arthritis have been tested and found to raise homocysteine. These include:

- Methotrexate[118]
- Corticosteroids[119]
- Sulphasalazine[120]

Some of these drugs are bad news as far as homocysteine is concerned because they knock out folate. Many studies have shown homocysteine levels to be raised in those patients treated with methotrexate,[121] with all of these studies supporting the use of folate supplementation to lower homocysteine levels. If you need to be on them, make sure your doctor is also giving you sufficient folate supplement (and make sure you take them at different times of the day). Also, following the H–Factor Diet (see pages 141–4) will help minimise the effects of these drugs on your homocysteine level.

MEASURING YOUR HOMOCYSTEINE

Your homocysteine level is easy to measure at home (see Resources, page 348). Homocysteine is measured in mmol/l. We used to think a 'high' level was above 15 units (mmol/l). At this level and above your risk of a heart attack increases and your Alzheimer's risk doubles. Now, however, levels as low as 7 units are being linked to increased disease risk. Basically, there's no official safe level and no guarantee that the diet and supplements you are currently taking are keeping homocysteine at bay. Up to 30 per cent of people with a history of heart disease have a homocysteine level above 14 units. The average level in Britain is 10.5. Experts believe that a level below 6 units is ideal. If you have any of the risk factors opposite it's especially important to get tested.

High homocysteine risk factors

These include:

- Genetic inheritance, meaning family history of heart disease, strokes, cancer, Alzheimer's disease, schizophrenia or diabetes
- Folate intake of less than 900mcg/day
- Increasing age
- Being male
- Oestrogen deficiency
- Excessive alcohol, coffee or tea intake
- Smoking
- Lack of exercise
- Hostility and repressed anger
- Inflammatory bowel diseases (coeliac, Crohn's, ulcerative colitis)
- *H. pylori*-generated ulcers
- Pregnancy
- Being a strict vegetarian or vegan
- High-fat diet with excessive red meat, high-fat dairy intake
- High salt intake

LOWERING YOUR HOMOCYSTEINE

The good news is that, whatever your homocysteine level is, you can lower it with the right combination of nutrients and dietary changes, together with lifestyle changes designed to reduce your risk. Follow the H-Factor Diet below.

The H-Factor Diet

Eat less fatty meat, more fish and vegetable protein
Have no more than four servings of lean meat a week;

continued

fish (but not fried) at least three times a week; and if you're not allergic or intolerant, a serving of a soya-based food, such as tofu, tempeh or soya sausages, or beans, such as kidney beans, chickpea hummus or baked beans, at least five times a week.

Eat your greens Have at least five servings of fruit or vegetables a day. This means eating two pieces of fruit every single day, and three servings of vegetables. Vary your selections from day to day. Make sure half of what's on your plate for each main meal is vegetables.

Have a clove of garlic a day Either eat a clove of garlic or take a garlic supplement every day. You can take garlic oil capsules or powdered garlic supplements.

Don't add salt to your food Miss out the salt while you're cooking and don't add it to the food on your plate. The only salt I consider healthy is Solo salt, which has half the sodium of ordinary salt and lots of potassium and magnesium. Use this in moderation instead.

Cut back on tea and coffee Don't drink more than one cup of caffeinated or decaffeinated coffee, or two cups of tea, in a day. Instead choose from the wide variety of herbal teas and grain coffees available.

Limit your alcohol Keep your alcohol intake to no more than half a pint of beer, or one glass of red wine, in a day. Ideally, limit your intake to two pints of beer or four glasses of wine a week.

Reduce your stress If you are under a lot of stress, or find yourself reacting stressfully much of the time, make a decision to reduce your stress load by changing both the circumstances that are causing you stress and your

continued

attitude. Simple additions to your life, such as yoga, meditation and/or exercise, or seeing a counsellor if you have some issues to resolve, can make all the difference.

Stop smoking If you smoke, make a decision to stop, and seek help to do it. There is simply no safe level of smoking as far as homocysteine and your health is concerned. Smoking is nothing less than slow suicide. The sooner you stop the longer you'll live.

Correct oestrogen deficiency If you are post-menopausal, or have menopausal symptoms or other menstrual irregularities, check your oestrogen and progesterone levels with a hormone saliva test. If you are oestrogen or progesterone deficient, you can correct this with 'natural progesterone' HRT in the form of a transdermal skin cream. Natural progesterone has none of the associated risks of HRT and your body can make its own oestrogen from progesterone.

Supplement a high-strength multivitamin every day
Take a high-strength multivitamin and mineral supplement providing at least 25mg of the main B vitamins, 200mcg of folate and 10mcg each of vitamins B_{12} and B_6, plus A, D and E, and the minerals magnesium, selenium, chromium and zinc. Also, supplement 1g of vitamin C for general health, as well as the specific homocysteine-lowering nutrients indicated below.

Take homocysteine supplements The most powerful and the quickest way to restore a normal H score – to below 6 units – is to supplement specific homocysteine-lowering nutrients. These include vitamins B_2, B_6, B_{12}, folic acid, tri-methyl glycine (TMG) and zinc. Here are the guidelines:

continued

Homocysteine-lowering nutrients

Nutrient	No risk below 6	Low risk 6–9	High risk 9–15	Very high risk above 15
Folate	200mcg	400mcg	1,200mcg	2,000mcg
B_{12}	10mcg	500mcg	1,000mcg	1,500mcg
B_6	25mg	50mg	75mg	100mg
B_2	10mg	15mg	20mg	50mg
Zinc	5mg	10mg	15mg	20mg
TMG	500mg	750mg	1.5–3g	3–6g

The current vogue is to recommend folic acid. However, this alone is far less effective than the correct nutrients in combination. The amount you need also depends on your current homocysteine level. One study found that homocysteine scores reduced by 17 per cent on high-dose folic acid alone, 19 per cent on vitamin B_{12} alone; 57 per cent on folic acid plus B_{12}; and 60 per cent on folic acid, B_{12} and B_6.[122] All this was achieved in three weeks!

However, even better results would have been achieved by including TMG. TMG is the best methyl 'donor' to supplement – better than SAMe. Some companies produce combinations of these nutrients (see Resources, page 350). These are the most cost-effective supplements for restoring a healthy homocysteine level.

The combination of the diet and supplements recommended above has the potential to halve your homocysteine score in weeks. The goal is to bring your score to below 6. Mine is 4.5. Your homocysteine score is probably the best objective measure of whether you are achieving optimum nutrition for you.

Dig deeper by reading my book, co-authored with Dr James Braly, *The H Factor*.

SUMMARY

- **Both vitamins B$_5$ (pantothenic acid) and B$_3$ (niacinamide) have been shown to help** arthritis sufferers. The best food sources are mushrooms, eggs and lentils for B$_5$ and turkey, chicken, tuna and mackerel for B$_3$. I recommend 500–1,000mg vitamin B$_5$ a day for arthritis sufferers for a trial period of two months. If this helps, reduce the dose and see if the benefit is maintained. If not, return to the higher dose. If there is no change in two months, return to the basic dose.
- **Vitamin B$_6$ can help control inflammation**. Good food sources include Brussels sprouts, bananas, red kidney beans and cauliflower. Or supplement 50mg per day, preferably as part of a multivitamin and mineral or vitamin B complex.
- **A combination of folic acid and vitamin B$_{12}$ has also helped arthritis sufferers**. The best food sources of folic acid are wheatgerm, spinach, broccoli and peanuts. The best food sources of vitamin B$_{12}$ are sardines, oysters and tuna. Appropriate daily doses would be 200mcg of folic acid and at least 10mcg of B$_{12}$ (500–1,000mcg if your homocysteine level is high).
- **If you have any of the associated risk factors for high homocysteine, have your level tested** and, if high, follow the H-Factor Diet and supplement recommendations in the chart on pages 141–4.

CHAPTER 12

STOP STRESSING YOUR JOINTS

A good way of viewing health is to consider that we exist on three levels: physical, chemical and psychological. If all three are in balance, disease is unlikely to occur. Good nutrition aims to bring the body's chemistry back into balance. This chapter and Chapters 13, 24, 25 and 26 are all about the physical side of arthritis.

Physical imbalance or strain will ultimately cause joint damage, however good your diet. So there is little point in improving your nutrition if you do nothing about the underlying causes of mechanical stress. In practical terms this means two things: identifying mechanical stresses and imbalances, and correcting them.

THE CAUSES OF JOINT STRAIN

Joint strain usually occurs for one or more of the following reasons. The first is one-off traumas or accidents. These may occur at any time in life, including childhood. A bad fall, a sports-related injury, a car accident or any other trauma can throw out the body's mechanics so that the musculature has to adapt to a new posture to compensate. But it cannot compensate forever, and the result may be joint strain, which can lead to arthritis.

Joint strain can also come about after small amounts of trauma over a long period of time, such as 'repetitive strain' actions in your occupation or sporting activities (for example, repetitive lifting of things in the wrong way, or typing while sitting in the wrong position). Then there are long-term postural factors to consider, such as how you sit, lie down, walk and move around. These too can induce strain over long periods of time. In fact, our posture and way of moving are the result of everything that has happened to us up until now, including injuries, accidents and occupations we have long forgotten. The body, however, never forgets.

Understanding the first signs

The first sign of mechanical imbalances is periodic pain – the odd back pain or joint pain. It is well worth paying attention to this, as it is a sign of the body registering discomfort. Pain itself can be seen as the body's way of protecting an area, in this case by encouraging you to inhibit movement – so arthritis could be seen as the body's way of immobilising joints that can no longer take any more strain.

The skeleton is much more than a mechanical structure. It is a storehouse of minerals, a factory for new cells and a protected conduit for nerves and blood vessels. From each spinal vertebra extends a nerve, vein and artery. If the spine is compressed, this will affect both the nerve and blood supply, not only to the spine itself, but also to other parts of the body which are under the control of these vital nerve signals and need a good blood supply to work optimally. Changes in the structure of the body will affect its function, which is why a wide variety of health problems can be the result of musculoskeletal imbalances.

IDENTIFYING AND CORRECTING
MECHANICAL IMBALANCES

Osteopathy can identify and correct mechanical imbalances, as can chiropractic and physiotherapy, and is an essential part of the proper treatment of all musculoskeletal diseases, including arthritis. These practitioners can identify what the problem is by palpation, by measuring and analysing how you move, and sometimes by X-ray. Palpation involves feeling the position of joints and the nature of the soft tissue (which includes ligaments, tendons and muscle), and an experienced practitioner learns much from it. The goal of these therapies is to increase your flexibility and your ability to adapt to different physical demands so that you can go about your life with the least strain. (To find your nearest practitioner, see Resources, page 344).

Corrections to joint structure can be made by working on soft tissue with massage techniques, and on bone alignment through manipulation. However, these treatments must be backed up by exercise, or corrections to mechanical behaviour, to maintain and improve mechanical function. If you improve movement within a joint, the blood supply and nerve function may also improve – helping it to heal faster.

Helping yourself

Although osteopaths, chiropractors and physiotherapists can point you in the right direction, your mechanical health depends mainly on what you do yourself. The first step is to increase your awareness of your body as a complex and incredible instrument. Begin to notice how you put it under stress. If you have weak or tense areas, you may benefit greatly from regular massage, regular check-ups and specific exercises. Mechanical health depends on regular exercise to maintain flexibility and strength. This is a vital part of your anti-arthritis programme and is covered in Chapter 26.

There are many other excellent exercises and techniques that can help re-educate your body, including the Alexander Technique, Feldenkrais, postural integration, hatha yoga and others. The Alexander Technique is a way of changing habitual reactions that, when repeated over many years, can cause joint trauma, and it helps to release tension in the body. Learning the Alexander Technique can help to change habitual patterns, thereby reducing the strain. It is generally more applicable in cases of osteoarthritis or traumatic arthritis, although it is useful in the early stages of rheumatoid arthritis. (To find your nearest teacher, see Resources, page 346.)

THE IMPORTANCE OF SITTING CORRECTLY

Most people spend a lot of time sitting and lying down. And the way you sit can make unnecessary demands on your muscles, strain your bones and ligaments, restrict your breathing, and impair your circulation.

Many office chairs are not designed for good sitting posture. However, there are some simple adjustments you can make that will reduce unnecessary stress. First of all, the chair you sit on needs to be the correct height for your work surface so that you don't have to slouch and collapse your spine and chest to do your work. You may need to increase the height or lower it. It is good to have your feet firmly on the floor, so if you are short, you may work best by putting something firm on the ground, like a couple of telephone directories, to rest your feet on.

Are you sitting comfortably?

1 When you are seated, make sure you sit straight on the sitting bones, which are the curved ridges of bone that you can feel at the base of the pelvis when sitting. If you sit on the sitting bones, your spine has more chance of being straight.

Often we slouch back, collapsing the spine and resting on the coccyx (tail bone).

2 Now check your eye position. If you get eye strain, you may well be getting joint and spine strain too. The eyes literally lead the nervous system. You will automatically adjust your body to see whatever you are working on. If you are too high you will strain forward. Experiment with changing the angle and height of material you are reading or, if you use a computer, the level of the screen in relation to you. If you are typing, alter the angle of the material you copy so that it is easy to read. Angled writing surfaces, such as old school desks, and angled copy-holders (like lecterns), help to reduce unnecessary strain.

3 Your arms also need to be in the correct position. Armchairs can encourage you to lift your shoulders to rest your arms

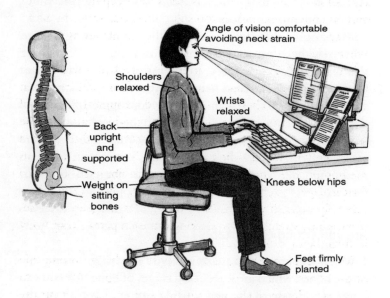

Figure 18 – Correct sitting position

on the arm of the chair. This creates unnecessary strain. Your shoulders should be down and back at all times. Check that your arms, elbows and wrists can remain flexible while you work so there is neither strain nor restricted circulation. Rest your hands in your lap when you are not working.

If you do spend a lot of time at a desk, it's worth getting an excellent book by Julie Friedberger called *Office Yoga* (see Recommended Reading). This book gives simple exercises that you can do to improve flexibility, which are good for anyone with arthritis.

THE DANGERS OF GOING TO BED

We spend up to a third of our lives lying down, so the position you lie in makes all the difference to your musculoskeletal system for two reasons. The first is that a bad sleeping position or certain conditions, such as too soft a mattress, strain the body. The second is that the spine and other joints are nourished when you are asleep.

During the day you get shorter. Between your spinal vertebrae are discs of cartilage that are softer than the cartilage at the end of bones. These get compressed through the action of gravity when you are standing or sitting, which shortens the space between the discs. When you lie down the discs expand and literally suck in nutrients from adjoining tissues. This method of receiving nutrients is called imbibition and is vital for cartilage, which has no direct blood supply. You can therefore help nourish your joints by doing loosening-up exercises (very gently stretching and shaking out each part of your body in turn) before going to bed.

Most people sleep in the foetal position, lying on one side or the other, with legs flexed. This is fine provided the surface is correct. However, too soft a mattress or too hard a mattress, too many or too few pillows can strain the spine and neck.

Generally speaking, the spine should be horizontal and straight and not unduly flexed up or down. Thus a soft mattress that allows the lower spine to sink, and too many pillows that allow the neck to flex upwards, will introduce strain. If you find it difficult to lie on your side this may be because of mechanical imbalances. It is also fine to sleep on your back, provided the surface you lie on is firm enough.

Sleep well with a specially designed mattress

If sleep is a problem because of back pain, you may benefit from a specially contoured mattress called Klass Vaki, which is Afrikaans for the 'Sandman'. It's made of foam of different densities that support the body in places where it wouldn't normally be touching the mattress. According to research reported in the *South African Medical Journal*, it's been found to reduce heart rate and allow back muscles to recover (see Resources, page 346).

An osteopath, chiropractor or physiotherapist can advise you about good mattresses and sleeping positions (see Resources, page 344).

REDUCING STRESS/THE PSYCHOLOGY OF ARTHRITIS

We all need some stimulation or we slide into apathy. Indeed, boredom can be stressful in itself. For many of us, however, 'over-stimulation', leading to excessive stress, is the problem. Since we all have different abilities to cope with different circumstances, each person has an optimal stress level at which they can function well.

In order to avoid excessive stress, it is important to understand its symptoms and causes. Stress – anger, fear, excitement, frustration – stimulates the adrenal glands. So do certain chemical substances, including refined sugar, salt, cigarettes, alcohol, tea and coffee. All these things, in excess, cause the same reaction.

WHAT STRESS DOES

The stress reaction is a physical one, for the very good reason that, when primitive man had feelings of stress, the cause was likely to be physical danger. His body's reactions prepared him to run away fast, or to turn and fight.

The adrenal glands therefore release adrenalin, which produces a 'high' almost like a drug. They also release cortisone. Together, these two hormones gear the whole body for action: digestion shuts down; glucose is released into the bloodstream to fuel the nerves and muscles; breathing, heart rate and blood pressure all increase, ready to deliver oxygen to the cells to burn the fuel and make energy.

TOO MUCH STRESS

If this process happens too often, side effects build up: nutrients are used up; digestion is slow and disrupted; resistance to infection declines; and minor problems occur, such as headaches, stiffness, insomnia or moodiness. If nothing is done, major problems can develop, such as heart disease, diabetes, arthritis and even cancer.

The adrenal glands can become exhausted from overstimulation. So can the thyroid, which works closely with the adrenals. A vicious circle is created whereby more and more stimulation is needed to get them working, so there may be cravings for harmful stimulants like sugar and coffee. As the systems become worn down, there may be weight gain, higher blood cholesterol, slower thinking and reduced energy.

Stress overload can be measured by determining a person's levels of two key stress hormones, cortisol and DHEA (a precursor for stress hormones). These are best measured in saliva and a standard stress test involves providing five saliva samples at different intervals over a 24-hour period. These are then sent for analysis. Such tests, available through nutritional therapists, can determine whether a person needs to pursue a nutritional or hormonal strategy to restore proper stress response. DHEA levels are often low in those with rheumatoid arthritis[123] and there is good reason to believe that, in such cases, supplementing 50mg or more of DHEA may help restore normal stress response, thus reducing inflammation.

ACTION AGAINST STRESS

In many stressful situations, the most we do is drum our fingers or make a rude remark, or, even worse, keep our feelings bottled up inside – which can lead to hidden resentment. Such responses do not use up the nutrients released into the blood, nor do they stimulate the physical mechanisms designed to burn them up.

This is one reason why exercise is important for people who are stressed in any way. Obviously it is best taken at the time of stress – a brisk walk or vigorous exercise session is good first aid. If that is impossible, you will benefit from regular exercise anyway.

How to relax

Simple relaxation techniques also help the body and mind to get back to normal.

Tense your muscles as hard as you can and then relax, starting with your feet and ending with your facial muscles. Or just clench your fists tightly and relax. Or take a deep breath, hold it for a count of ten, and breathe it all out at once. Yoga breathing and meditation exercises are also excellent de-stressors.

Long-term stress control

What you really need is to counter stress at source. Try the following suggestions:

- Limit your working hours to, at most, ten a day, five days a week. And always have a proper lunch break – at least 30 minutes and preferably an hour.
- Keep at least one and a half days a week completely free of routine work.
- Use this free time to cultivate a relaxing hobby, do something creative or take exercise, preferably in the fresh air.
- Adopt a relaxed manner. For instance, walk and talk more slowly. If you find this difficult, try acting as 'if' you were a relaxed person, almost as a game.
- Avoid obvious pressures, such as taking on too many commitments. Learn to say 'no', or 'not now'.
- Learn to see when a problem is somebody else's responsibility and refuse to take it on.
- If you have an emotional problem you cannot solve alone, seek advice.
- Concentrate on one task at a time, and focus all your attention on the present.
- Learn to say what is on your mind instead of suppressing it. You don't have to be aggressive – just state your point of view clearly and truthfully.
- Listen to what other people say to you, and about you.
- Look long and hard at all the stresses in your life. Make a list of them. Try to take a positive attitude to things that can't be changed. If change is possible – take action. Don't let things wear you down.

There is more information on how to deal with stress in my book *Beat Stress and Fatigue* (see Recommended Reading).

CHAPTER 13

THE HEALING POWER
OF WATER

Water is the most important nutrient for the human body. Your body is 65 per cent water. Although you can survive for a month without food, after a few days without water you would die. Water, which is made up of hydrogen and oxygen (H_2O), has remarkable properties. It can store, absorb and transmit heat very effectively – as ice, water or steam. It is also remarkably non-toxic and can therefore be used internally and externally (although there is an anecdotal story of a man who died after drinking 3 litres/5¼ pints of water in 20 minutes, showing that almost everything is toxic, depending on the dose). It has been used therapeutically for thousands of years by cultures all over the world. In India, for example, the *Rig Veda*, thought to have been written about 1500 BC, states that, 'Water cures the fever's glow'. Hippocrates used water treatments extensively around 400 BC. He wrote, 'For the bath soothes pain in the side, chest and back; cuts the sputum, promotes expectoration, improves the respiration, and allays lassitude; for it soothes the joints and outer skin ...'

THE BENEFITS OF HYDROTHERAPY

Hydrotherapy means the use of water in any form for the maintenance of health or the treatment of disease. At different times in history hydrotherapy has been popular. It is a common naturopathic technique in Germany, but not so well-known in the UK, and there are still differing opinions as to its usefulness. A 1983 review of research suggested that its benefits were limited to external effects, helping to reduce pain but not changing the underlying basis of disease. Yet an article in a German medical journal reported that after hydrotherapy there were increased concentrations of immune complexes not seen in control patients who were not receiving hydrotherapy.[124]

Hydrotherapy and arthritis

Whether or not hydrotherapy can improve immune function, it is a very useful and safe method for reducing localised pain and inflammation and improving circulation. Exposing an inflamed area to cold water has a depressant, calming effect and may be a useful way of calming down inflamed joints. If, however, the temperature is too cold (for example in the case of ice compresses), there is a stimulating rather than a calming reaction, which is not desirable for an actively inflamed and hot area.

On the other hand, stimulating the blood flow to a joint is generally beneficial: it helps to remove toxins and improve the supply of nutrients, as well as stimulating the movement of fluid within joints needed to nourish the cartilage. Improving circulation to a joint is best achieved by alternating hot and cold, usually in the form of compresses.

COMPRESSES

Two simple procedures may be helpful in treating arthritis. The first is the cold compress. This can help to calm down joints that are actively inflamed and hot. If you are slightly feverish as well, this is a good indication that a cold compress is suitable.

1 Put cold water and ice into a bowl of water. The temperature should be between 13°C and 18°C (55°F and 65°F). In other words, it should feel cold but not so cold that it hurts or numbs you.
2 Soak a towel in this water, wring it out, and place it on the affected area. You will need to soak and wring out the towel every two or three minutes to maintain the cold temperature.
3 Do this for about ten minutes, then dry the area.

The cold compress should reduce pain and inflammation, which may be particularly useful in rheumatoid arthritis, gout, bursitis, tendonitis and tenosynovitis. If the water is much too cold, the body can react to this by heating up the joint instead. So be careful to get the temperature right. You'll soon find out what works for you.

Movement through heat and cold

Alternating hot and cold compresses are used to improve circulation to a joint or area of the body that has become congested. Often, arthritic joints have little movement and poor circulation. Heat improves circulation and flexibility. So does extreme cold, by causing a heating reaction. This combination may help to get nutrients to the joints, and toxic material away, and has been shown to increase blood flow to extremities by 95 per cent.[125] There are differing views about the length of each phase. I recommend you try a hot compress for three minutes, followed by a cold compress for 30–60 seconds, and repeat this three times, as follows:

1 Make a bowl of hot water (about 37–40°C or 98–104°F), hot enough to produce skin redness if prolonged, but not so hot that you have to take your hand out.

continued

2   Soak a towel in this, and wring it out, then apply it to the affected area. Leave for 3 minutes.
3   Meanwhile, soak another towel in cold water, wring that out and wrap it around ice cubes, which will help to keep the towel very cold.
4   Apply this after the 3 minutes has elapsed, and leave for 30–60 seconds.

If you prefer, use an ice pack instead of the cold compress.

Caution Check the water temperature with a thermometer the first time you try these compresses. If you are diabetic, do not use the hot/cold compress without your doctor or naturopath's permission. Naturopaths are fully trained in hydrotherapy techniques, many of which are more advanced than those I have described. Should you wish to explore this avenue further I recommend you consult a naturopath. (To find your nearest practitioner, see Resources, page 344).

THERAPEUTIC BATHS

Another useful way of stimulating circulation is to have a cold shower after a hot bath or shower. If you are trying to stimulate circulation in a particular area, shower this area with cold water for just long enough to cool the area down. Your body will respond by warming it up, leaving you with a healthy glow after the shower. This is particularly good before an exercise session, as part of your warm-up.

After an exercise session you might benefit from a bath containing sodium bicarbonate. This makes the water and the skin more alkaline (less acidic) and is said to help the body detoxify. After therapeutic massage, or exercise, there can be a build-up of acid end products of metabolism. Drinking a glass of water containing sodium bicarbonate (such as Eno) and having a warm bath with 100g (3½oz) of sodium bicarbonate in it is thought to help reduce stiffness. Sodium bicarbonate is the same thing as bicarbonate of soda (used to bake cakes) – it's very inexpensive. Eno can be bought in sachets to drink with water after an exercise session or a therapeutic massage.

Water exercises

As well as its heating and cooling effects, water provides resistance to the body, which in itself improves the flow of fluid within joints. Water pressure (provided by showers or Jacuzzis) is particularly good for this. Water also provides extra resistance, which makes it the ideal medium for exercising in without straining the joints. Many exercises for arthritis can be practised in water, and some can even be done in the bath. At least one weekly session of exercise in water is advisable for any kind of arthritic condition.

PART 3

REBUILDING YOUR JOINTS

CHAPTER 14

BALANCE YOUR BONE-BUILDING NUTRIENTS

There are many bone-building nutrients that are essential to bone health. Although the key players are calcium and magnesium, there are many other minerals that have been shown to play a role, including boron, zinc, copper, manganese and phosphorus as well as vitamins C, D, K, B_6 and folic acid. This chapter covers mainly calcium, magnesium, vitamin D and boron, since the remaining nutrients are covered in other chapters.

THE MAJOR MINERAL: CALCIUM

Calcium is the most abundant mineral in the body, accounting for 1.6 per cent of our body mass. Of the 1,200g calcium in our body, more than 99 per cent is in our bones and teeth. The remainder is present in our muscles, nerves and bloodstream, where it plays a crucial role in many enzymes and in the production of nerve signals and muscular energy.

Calcium is relatively well absorbed, with an average of 30 per cent of ingested calcium reaching the bloodstream. But its absorption into the bloodstream depends on many factors. An excess of alcohol, a lack of hydrochloric acid in the stomach, or an excess of acid–forming foods (mainly protein) can decrease its absorption, as does the presence of lead and other toxic minerals, which compete with it for absorption sites.

A hormone produced by the parathyroid gland – parathormone (PTH) – helps the absorption of calcium. It does this by converting vitamin D into another hormone that makes the gut wall more permeable to calcium. So, a lack of vitamin D is another factor to consider. PTH also helps to keep calcium in circulation once it has been absorbed, by reducing excretion of calcium via the kidneys.

Once in the body, there are many factors that influence calcium balance. Once again, heavy metals (such as lead) compete with calcium. So do sodium (salt), tea, cocoa and red wine. In post-menopausal women, the low levels of oestrogen

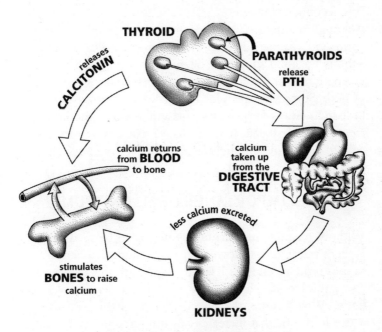

Figure 19 – Calcium balance

also make calcium less retainable. One of the greatest factors in calcium balance is exercise or, rather, lack of it. Studies at NASA, where they discovered losses of calcium in astronauts living in zero gravity conditions, showed that weight-bearing exercise (such as walking) can raise calcium levels in the body by 2 per cent or more.[1]

Once in the body, calcium is constantly moving from blood to bone. It is released into the blood when it is needed to stimulate muscles or nerves. Once this reaction is over, the thyroid gland recalls calcium to the bones by secreting the hormone calcitonin. An imbalance in the thyroid or parathyroid gland can also interfere with calcium balance.

Important minerals in the diet

Bones contain magnesium and phosphorus, as well as calcium. Although phosphorus is abundant in most people's diets, calcium and magnesium are often deficient. Dairy produce, although a good source of calcium, is not a good source of magnesium. Nuts, seeds and root vegetables are good sources of both. Since most people's diets contain dairy produce, but little in the way of vegetables, nuts and seeds, magnesium deficiency is widespread. It is estimated that fewer than 20 per cent of people get enough magnesium.[2]

THE IMPORTANCE OF MAGNESIUM

Without magnesium, calcium is unlikely to be used properly. Recent research has shown that magnesium-deficient infants cannot produce enough PTH to respond to low calcium levels in the blood, which results in calcium deficiency in the body.[3] What's more, the conversion of vitamin D into the active hormone that increases calcium retention is dependent on magnesium. In order to be incorporated into bone, calcium forms crystals (another process facilitated by an enzyme that is magnesium-dependent).[4]

Low magnesium levels are associated with osteoporosis, and research by Dr Guy Abraham has shown remarkable results in reversing osteoporosis using a multi-nutrient approach including magnesium.[5] He studied 26 post-menopausal women all receiving hormone-replacement therapy. All the women had their bone density assessed. Seven patients received dietary advice similar to that recommended in this book, whereas 19 received the same dietary advice and six nutritional supplements. These provided a broad spectrum of vitamins and minerals, including 500mg of calcium and 600mg of magnesium.

On their return visits, six to 12 months later, bone density was measured again. Those with dietary advice and hormone replacement therapy had an insignificant 0.7 per cent increase in bone density, whereas those also taking supplements had a 16 times greater increase in bone density of 11 per cent. At the start of the study, 15 out of the 19 women due to take supplements had a bone density below the fracture threshold, indicating osteoporosis. Within a year of taking supplements only seven patients still had bone densities below this threshold. This study shows, without a doubt, how potent a combined intake of vitamins and minerals is for reversing bone disease, in comparison with standard drug treatment.

Magnesium is also important in an increasingly common problem called fibromyalgia (see Chapter 18). This is a condition in which muscles throughout the body become stiff and painful – it is increasingly common, particularly among older women. One theory is that it is due to a defect in energy production within muscle cells, leading to a build-up of the wrong chemicals, causing muscle pain and stiffness. In pilot trials, magnesium malate (magnesium plus malic acid, both of which are needed for proper energy production) has been shown to produce good results.

VITAMIN D

As I've already mentioned, vitamin D is needed to enable calcium to be used properly by the body. It is converted into a hormone, calcitriol, which works with PTH to control calcium balance in the body. Calcitriol also plays an important role in the immune system, because it is able to suppress the pro-inflammatory chemicals I talked about in Chapter 3, and enhance the anti-inflammatory ones. High doses of vitamin D have been found to reduce pain and modify disease.[6]

Healthy sun

Vitamin D can be made in the skin, in the presence of sunlight, which may be one reason why arthritis sufferers often feel better in the summer. How much vitamin D you need varies with age, weight, percentage of body fat, where you live in the world (latitude), colour of your skin, time of year, use of sunblock, and your level of sun exposure. The amount you need from diet depends on the amount you produce in your skin. Vitamin D production is apparently at its highest in the autumn, perhaps as an evolutionary adaptation to store it up for the winter months ahead.

Getting enough vitamin D

The low vitamin D intake in several European countries is due to the fact that only a few foods are naturally good sources of vitamin D.[7] Fatty fish such as herring, mackerel, pilchards, sardines and tuna, as well as eggs, are rich sources. There's a little in milk, meat and fortified foods. If you eat these foods regularly *and* expose yourself to natural daylight for half an hour a day, you will achieve the equivalent of about 15mcg (600iu). The ideal intake is at least 30mcg, so supplement an additional 15mcg of vitamin D each day. A good multivitamin may provide this. Although supplementing vitamin D on its own is not effective for increasing bone density in osteoporosis, it is effective when combined with calcium and other nutrients.[8] Supplementing the active hormone calcitriol is the most effective of all.[9] This suggests that people with osteoporosis, and perhaps arthritis, have difficulty converting vitamin D into the active hormone calcitriol. Widespread magnesium deficiency is one factor that could account for this.

A common deficiency

Vitamin D deficiency among the elderly is far from uncommon. According to a survey published in the *New England Journal of Medicine*, 57 per cent of 290 senior citizens in hospital had low blood levels of this bone-building vitamin.[10] In 2005, a group from Minnesota found that 100 per cent of elderly patients admitted for fragility fractures were vitamin D deficient, despite the fact that half of them were taking vitamin D supplements.[11]

It is not just the elderly who are at risk. At least 60 per cent of the adult population in the UK do not get enough vitamin D according to the National Diet and Nutrition Survey for 1995–2004. This survey also showed that 12 per cent were actually deficient. Vitamin D inadequacy is common among post-menopausal women,[12] vegetarians, those eating low-fat diets, and those not getting enough sunlight (see Chapter 15).

Another issue is that current recommended levels of vitamin D are thought to be too low and experts say there is an urgent need to recommend an intake of vitamin D that is effective.[13] According to Reinhold Vieth, professor of nutritional sciences at Toronto University, 'Current dietary guidelines for vitamin D in the UK are incorrect in stating that adults below age 50 require no vitamin D and specify too little for older people. Sun avoidance advice makes the vitamin D problem even worse in the UK. The result is an unacceptably high occurrence of what should be regarded as toxic vitamin D deficiency.'

Preventing arthritis through vitamin D

There is evidence from clinical trials that high-dose vitamin D (1,000–2,000iu, or 25–50mcg vitamin D per day) can prevent many diseases including arthritis. According to Michael Holick, considered to be the world's leading expert on vitamin D, women can reduce their risk of rheumatoid arthritis by about 44 per cent if they ensure their daily intake of vitamin D is at least 400iu.[14] The average UK diet will provide about 150iu of vitamin D per day.

Osteoarthritis develops more frequently and progresses more rapidly in patients who are vitamin D deficient. Vitamin D deficiency is alarmingly common in patients with musculoskeletal pain[15] and treatment of patients with back pain with high dose vitamin D resulted in alleviation of pain in almost 100 per cent of patients.[16]

CALCIUM: HOW SUPPLEMENTS CAN HELP

In summary, the body can use calcium better, helping to make strong bones and joints, if your diet also provides adequate amounts of magnesium and vitamin D. Supplementing an extra 500mg of calcium and magnesium, plus at least 15mcg (600iu) to 30mcg (1200iu) of vitamin D is likely to offer optimal protection for bones and joints. If exposure to sunlight is limited, Dr Holick maintains that a minimum of 1,000iu per day from food and/or supplements is required to maintain a healthy concentration in the blood.[17]

BORON FOR HEALTHY BONES

The trace element boron is abundant in soil, food and in humans. Most people consume about 3mg a day, mainly from

vegetables. High levels tend to be found in apples, pears, tomatoes, soya, prunes, raisins, dates and honey. Boron is an essential element for plants, possibly because it helps control plant
growth hormones.

Although it has not yet been conclusively proven as
essential, boron is found in the human body and does appear
to be both bioactive and beneficial.[18] It appears to be more
concentrated in the thyroid and parathyroid glands, which
might suggest a role in their function. Animal studies point
to an interaction between boron and calcium balance. Deficiency of vitamin D increases the need for boron, and it is
suspected that boron is somehow involved with the action
of the parathyroid hormone, which helps maintain calcium
within bone. Animals given boron supplements were found
to be much less susceptible to the effects of magnesium
deficiency. In plants, boron is involved with the transport of
calcium.

BORON AND ARTHRITIS

Although only one properly controlled double-blind trial has
been published, there have been many reports linking boron
with arthritis. Dr Newnham, working in New Zealand,
reported the successful treatment of rheumatoid arthritis with
low doses of boron.[19] He noted that areas with low levels of
boron in the soil, such as Mauritius and Jamaica, had high inci-
dences of arthritis, whereas areas with high boron soil levels,
such as Israel, had a very low incidence of arthritis. He
reported that supplementing 6–9mg of boron per day
improved symptoms within a few weeks in 80–90 per cent of
cases. He has also shown that boron supplementation can
completely cure arthritis in horses, cattle and dogs. In addition,
Dr Neil Ward, from the University of Surrey, found lower levels of boron in the bones of rheumatoid arthritis sufferers
compared with those without arthritis.[20]

In the late 1980s Dr Neilson and colleagues from the US Department of Agriculture investigated boron in relation to mineral and hormone balance in post-menopausal women.[21] They found that supplementing 3mg a day helped the body to retain calcium and magnesium, especially in those with poor magnesium status. It also increased the levels of the hormones testosterone and oestradiol (in relation to oestrogen), which is the only agent so far tested that consistently increases bone density in post-menopausal women. According to Dr Neilson, 'The findings suggest that supplementation of a low-level diet with an amount of boron commonly found in diets high in fruits and vegetables induces changes in post-menopausal women consistent with the prevention of calcium loss and bone demineralisation.'

In 1990 the first double-blind trial on boron and arthritis was conducted.[22] Ten arthritic patients were placed on boron (6mg) and ten on placebo pills. Of the ten on boron, five improved, whereas only one improved on the placebo. There were no side effects.

According to Professor Bryce-Smith, who has researched boron extensively, there is now a considerable body of scientific evidence pointing to boron as a beneficial factor in the metabolism of animals and humans. Both osteoporosis and rheumatoid arthritis are associated with a boron deficiency. He says that the current evidence indicates supplementing 3mg of boron a day could help prevent and treat structural disorders in bones in both men and post-menopausal women, with little risk of side effects. Further scientific and medical studies are certainly needed in this area.

Getting enough boron

These early studies of boron used daily supplements of 3–9mg, given as sodium borate. At much higher levels boron becomes toxic, as do most minerals. Some supplements now combine calcium, or calcium and magnesium, with boron. It would appear that supplementing up to 3mg a day, together with a high fruit and vegetable diet, would provide more than optimal intakes of this potentially important trace element.

See Chapter 23 for more about supplements.

SUMMARY

- **Although the most well-known bone-building nutrients** are calcium and vitamin D, other nutrients are necessary for healthy bones, including magnesium, phosphorus and boron. Whereas phosphorus is abundant in most people's diets, calcium and magnesium are often deficient.
- **Nuts, seeds and root vegetables** are good sources of both calcium and magnesium. Appropriate doses for supplementing are 300–600mg of both calcium and magnesium. Magnesium malate (magnesium plus malic acid) is also helpful for fibromyalgia (see Chapter 18).
- **Vitamin D** is needed to enable calcium to be used properly by the body. Good food sources include oily fish such as herring, mackerel, pilchards, sardines and tuna, as well as eggs. Eating these foods regularly and getting sufficient exposure to sunlight will give you the equivalent of about 15mcg (600iu). The ideal intake is at least 30mcg, so supplement an additional 15mcg of vitamin D daily. A good multivitamin may provide this. It should be supplemented with calcium and other nutrients.
- **Boron** is an essential element in plants, involved with the transport of calcium and thought to help control plant growth hormones. In humans it is thought to help the body retain calcium and magnesium and has been shown to improve arthritis symptoms. Good food sources include most vegetables, apples, pears, tomatoes, soya, prunes,

continued

raisins, dates and honey. I recommend supplementing up to 3mg a day, together with a high fruit and vegetable diet, to ensure optimal intake of this potentially important trace element.

CHAPTER 15

LIGHT – THE FORGOTTEN NUTRIENT

Research into light is still in its infancy, but we know that it is an essential nutrient for both the mind and body. We take in light in two ways: through the skin and through the eyes. Both stimulate glands in the body and affect hormone levels.

The whole chemistry of our bodies is designed around these stimulating effects of light. For example, the reason you wake up is that light, entering through the translucent portions of the skull, stimulates both the pineal and pituitary gland in the brain, which leads to increased adrenalin levels, to allow you to wake up full of energy. However, if you sleep with thick curtains drawn to exclude all natural light, and wake to the sound of an alarm clock, your body and mind are unnaturally jolted into wakefulness and are therefore unlikely to function at their best.

The skin has a layer of cells that contain melanin, a dark pigment. Melanin filters out solar radiation very effectively. Africans, who have very high melanin levels, filter out 50–95 per cent of solar radiation. This adaptation may serve two purposes: firstly it protects the skin from the oxidative effects of radiation responsible for the high skin cancer rate in white-skinned people living in hot countries; secondly it limits the amount of vitamin D made in the skin, probably in order to prevent toxicity.

THE SUNSHINE VITAMIN

John Ott, now a leading expert on the importance of light, noticed in his previous job, as a time-lapse photographer for Walt Disney, that flowers responded differently under different lighting conditions. One of his specialities was photographing flowers from bud to blossom. Yet, under certain lights, flowers wouldn't bloom or fertilise. He now believes that we benefit from a full spectrum of light wavelengths, supplied by the sun but not by most artificial light.

John Ott says that full-spectrum light must enter the eye and advocates that we should all spend some time outdoors in direct light, without glasses or contact lenses, which obscure the beneficial effect. He noticed that his arthritis improved when he started to spend time outdoors without glasses. Immunologist Jennifer Meek is convinced that even as little as three minutes of light entering the eye stimulates the immune system – which is under attack in arthritis.

Probably the most important effect of light is that it converts two chemicals, ergosterol and 7-dehydrocholesterol – found in layers of the skin – into vitamin D, the so-called 'sunshine vitamin'.

Getting enough sunlight

Modern life keeps us indoors away from the sun, which supplies 90 per cent of the vitamin D we need. A billion or more people in Europe obtain insufficient sunlight and vitamin D, putting them at increased risk of diabetes, high blood pressure, arthritis, multiple sclerosis, diseases of the bone and many of the common cancers. In fact, some experts believe that the epidemic of chronic disease caused by a lack of vitamin D is probably as large as the epidemics caused by smoking and obesity, but the importance is still not properly recognised by governments.

High-risk groups

'People who do not get adequate sunlight will have reduced formation in the skin of vitamin D_2 and D_3, rendering them vitamin D deficient if they are also not absorbing adequate vitamin D in the diet,' says Dr Stephen Davies, who identifies dark-skinned people living in northern climates as particularly at risk.

Others at risk include elderly housebound people, adults who work indoors all day, people living in urban northerly regions, and immigrants who rarely expose their skin to sunlight. So, for example, an Indian, who has dark skin and remains covered up much of the time, and is vegan (eating no meat, eggs or dairy products), is at risk of vitamin D deficiency. This causes rickets (in children) and osteomalacia (in adults) – diseases in which the bones become malleable. People with dark skin – no doubt due to their high melanin content – are most susceptible to rickets. Even if you do get enough calcium, a lack of UV radiation significantly impairs the body's utilisation of it.

A recent conference was held at the House of Commons to address the issue of 'sunlight, vitamin D and health' and addressed the issue of sun safety, pointing out that those regularly using sunscreen at factor 8 or above or avoiding sunshine were putting themselves at risk of vitamin D deficiency. This includes women who regularly use foundation cosmetics containing sunscreen.[23] Their advice is to sunbathe safely (without burning) at every opportunity, without using sunscreens. Safely means starting slowly (2–3 minutes each side) and gradually increasing from day to day.

When supplements might help

If you are mainly vegetarian and don't eat vitamin D-enriched foods, eggs or dairy produce, and do not get substantial exposure to sunlight, I would recommend supplementing your diet with 15mcg (600iu) of vitamin D daily. This level is found in many multivitamins and also in some calcium and magnesium supplements. If you live in a hot country and are exposed to substantial amounts of sunlight, be careful that you are not getting too much dietary vitamin D, because an excess has a negative effect on calcium balance.

LIGHT IN THE DARKNESS

When light enters the eye it stimulates the brain, which in turn shuts off melatonin production in the pineal gland. Melatonin, which is produced only in the absence of light, is one brain chemical that makes you sleepy. Its role in sleep problems, jet lag and depression is currently being researched.

A proportion of people suffering from depression have what is called seasonal affective disorder, or SAD. Dr Norman Rosenthal, from the US National Institutes of Health, wondered whether this might be to do with the length of exposure to daylight. As the days get shorter, these people get more depressed. To test this theory, he exposed volunteers to full-spectrum light equivalent to sunlight for up to three hours before dawn and after dusk. A control group had to follow the same routine but were exposed to dimmer lighting, equivalent to domestic lighting. While the dim lights made no difference, all 13 of the SAD patients exposed to full-spectrum lighting improved – some dramatically. Most found that they could once again cope with life and function in their jobs, whereas before they often entered a state of severe depression in the winter months.

Light and arthritis

Although I am aware of no studies that have examined the effects of light on arthritis, the beneficial effects of living in a sunnier climate have been reported by many arthritis sufferers. On the basis of the evidence above, especially if your arthritis and/or state of mind definitely get worse in the late winter and early spring, you may benefit from more direct exposure to full-spectrum light. You can achieve this by: spending more time outside, without glasses or contact lenses; taking a winter holiday in a sunny climate (especially between January and March when levels are at their lowest); and fitting full-spectrum lighting in the main rooms you live and work in.

See Chapter 23 for more about supplements.

SUMMARY

- **Spend more time outside**, without glasses or contact lenses.
- **Take a winter holiday in a sunny climate** (especially between January and March when levels are at their lowest).
- **Fit full-spectrum lighting in the main rooms you live and work in**.
- **If you are in the 'at risk' category** (elderly housebound people, adults who work indoors all day, people living in urban northerly regions, and immigrants who rarely expose their skin to sunlight), follow the advice regarding vitamin D in the previous chapter.

CHAPTER 16

THE CARTILAGE CONNECTION

The fact that some individuals develop arthritis at an early age, that it is more common in women, and that it can strike whole families, strongly suggests that something other than 'wear and tear' is involved. It is reasonable to consider that people may differ in their ability to regenerate healthy cartilage, since it is the degeneration of cartilage that seems to herald the beginning of osteoarthritis, the most common form of arthritis. Osteoarthritis sufferers do appear to have cartilage that is different in composition from that of non-sufferers.[24]

Believe it or not, you can rebuild cartilage. When the body goes into a state of inflammation and is trying to immobilise a damaged joint, it actually causes more and more damage to the cartilage, especially if the joint in question is a weight-bearing joint, such as the knees, hips or lower back. But you can rebuild it, as Ed Smith found out. You may remember Ed from Chapter 4; here is a brief reminder:

Case Study: Ed

Ed had always kept himself fit, by playing tennis and running, but started to experience joint pain in his mid-thirties and had operations on both knees to repair damage to the cartilage. By his mid-forties he was suffering from severe arthritis, with ever-increasing pain, and began to take a variety of anti-inflammatory drugs, but his knees just got worse, giving him excruciating pain after playing golf, his favourite leisure pursuit.

When I met him he was aged 57 and could barely walk without pain, let alone pursue his passion for golf. I told him to read and follow the earlier edition of this book, and gave him a list of supplements to take; this included 1.5g of glucosamine, essential fats, high dose niacinamide (500mg) and pantothenic acid (1,000mg), 3g of vitamin C, 250mg (400iu) of vitamin E and a high-potency multivitamin.

He did everything recommended in the book and took the supplements religiously every day. Although there was little improvement in the first two months, by the third month his knees were feeling better. By six months he was virtually pain-free.

'I would never have believed my pain could be reduced by such a large degree, and not return, no matter how much activity I do in a day or week.'

Five years on, Ed remains 95 per cent pain-free and has had no return or worsening of his symptoms – and he needs no medication. He regularly plays golf. I've switched him over to a daily nutrition supplement pack, which contains vitamins C and E, omega-3 and 6 oils, antioxidants and B vitamins. I am also giving him 1,500mg glucosamine hydrochloride with MSM and a combination of the herbs boswellia, hop extract and olive pulp extract, which is a superb antioxidant. I find these to be the most effective remedies for promoting comfortable joints, together with a healthy diet, low in meat and dairy produce, and high in fish, flax seeds, fruit and vegetables.

Ed is living proof that the body can heal itself if you give it the right nutrients. Vital for rebuilding are glucosamine and

MSM, a form of sulphur. In order to understand how they work, it helps to know what cartilage actually is.

WHAT IS CARTILAGE?

Cartilage is what we often call 'gristle' – the Adam's apple, the tip of the nose, the bone ends, and the shock absorbers between spinal vertebrae are all made of cartilage. It is a tough, elastic, translucent material. The kind of cartilage found at bone ends, fibrocartilage, is the strongest of all.

In foetal development, cartilage forms the framework for the body, and it then becomes calcified to produce bones. The bones of children are more pliable because they contain more cartilage and less calcium. At the tops of bones are regions called 'growth plates', where the cartilage develops, allowing bones to grow. Once calcification of cartilage has occurred, it cannot be reversed.

Cells that produce cartilage are called chondrocytes. Cartilage is made of collagen and proteoglycans (a complex of protein and carbohydrate), which together act as a kind of intercellular glue or cement. This complex is what is thought to give cartilage its special properties. Bone formation requires both the 'cement' (collagen and proteoglycans) and the 'bricks' (principally calcium and phosphorus), which combine into a compound known as hydroxyapatite.

What makes healthy cartilage?

Much research has focused on ways of improving the body's ability to make healthy cartilage and heal joints. To this end, green-lipped mussels have entered the repertoire of arthritis remedies. As bizarre as this may sound, there are good reasons for it. The green-lipped mussel contains high levels of protein, vitamins and minerals, and a type of proteoglycan, which is a natural joint lubricant and component of all cartilage. Glucosamine and chondroitin (a jelly-like substance that provides support and adhesiveness in bone, cartilage and skin) have also become popular, effective supplements for people with arthritis.

The theory, in accordance with the basic principle of optimum nutrition, is that if you provide your body cells with the materials they need to do their job properly, they will. If arthritis sufferers lack the necessary components to make healthy cartilage, why not provide what's needed? It is more likely to help than giving drugs that suppress the symptoms but do nothing to stop the disease. Unlike other body tissue, cartilage has no blood or nerve supply. It receives nutrients from the bodily fluid that is moved around joint spaces by compression and relaxation. Thus, exercise is a good way of improving nutrient transport to cartilage. During the day, the cartilaginous discs between our spinal vertebrae compress. At night, when we lie down, these discs expand, sucking in nutrients from surrounding body fluids.

THE TRUTH ABOUT GLUCOSAMINE AND CHONDROITIN

One of the best-known non-drug treatments for joint pain is glucosamine, an essential part of the building material for joints and the cellular 'glue' that holds the entire body together. It is a naturally occurring amino sugar (a molecule combining an amino acid with a simple sugar) and found in almost all the tissues of your body, although joint cartilage contains a higher concentration of glucosamine than any other structural tissue.[25] It is used to make N-acetylglucosamine, which, in turn, is one of the building blocks for making cartilage.

Daily wear and tear on our joints means that the connective tissue that surrounds them (cartilage, tendons and ligaments) requires constant renewal, needing an ongoing supply of glucosamine. Unfortunately, it appears that some people are less able to make glucosamine as they get older. When this rebuilding process slows down, the result is degenerative joint diseases such as arthritis.

The mechanism by which glucosamine appears to stop or reverse joint degeneration is by providing the body with the materials needed to build and repair cartilage. It plays a fundamental role in the formation of joints, tendons, ligaments, synovial fluid, bone and many more parts of the body, including the skin and blood vessels. Cartilage in joints consists of cells embedded in collagen that sits within a framework of watery proteoglycan gel. When this structure is working correctly, joints remain flexible and able to resist the pressure of impact and gravity. So glucosamine appears to stop or reverse joint degeneration by providing the body with the materials it needs to form these proteoglycans (the framework for joint structure) and may prevent their breakdown in the body.[26] There is also some evidence that glucosamine helps the incorporation of sulphur into cartilage (sulphur is an essential nutrient for keeping all connective tissue stable).[27]

Is your body making enough?

Although the body can make glucosamine, if you've got damaged joints you are unlikely to make enough – unless you are in the habit of munching on sea shells, which are the richest dietary source. Taking a substantial quantity of glucosamine as a nutritional supplement has been shown to slow down or even reverse this degenerative process. There are about 440,000 joint replacements every year in the US, and many could be avoided with the right nutrition. But how does glucosamine do the job?

Cartilage protection

Glucosamine appears to be particularly effective in protecting and strengthening the cartilage around your knees, hips, spine and hands. And although it can do little to actually restore cartilage that has completely worn away, it helps to prevent further joint damage and appears to slow the development of mild to moderate osteoarthritis. As mentioned earlier, traditional NSAIDs prescribed for arthritis actually impair your body's cartilage-building capacity.

A 2001 study in the *Lancet* reported that glucosamine actually slowed the progression of osteoarthritis of the knee.[28] Over the course of three years, they measured spaces between the patients' joints and tracked their symptoms. Those on glucosamine showed no further narrowing of joints in the knee, which is an indicator of thinning cartilage. Put another way, glucosamine appeared to protect the shock-absorbing cartilage that cushions the bones. In contrast, the condition of the patients taking the placebo steadily worsened.

Speedier healing

Because glucosamine helps to reinforce the cartilage around your joints, it may hasten the healing of acute joint injuries, such as sprained ankles or fingers, and of muscle injuries such as strains. In strengthening joints, glucosamine also helps to prevent future injury.

Back pain control

Glucosamine strengthens the tissues supporting the spinal discs that line the back. It may therefore improve back pain resulting from either muscle strain or arthritis, and speed the healing of strained back muscles. Glucosamine seems to have similar effects on pain in the upper spine and neck.

Healthier ageing

As your body ages, the cartilage supporting and cushioning all of your joints tends to wear down. By protecting and strengthening your cartilage, glucosamine may help to post-pone this process and reduce the risk of osteoarthritis.

Other benefits

Most studies indicate that arthritis sufferers can move more freely and report increased overall mobility after taking glucosamine. In addition, several studies have shown that glucosamine can be as effective as NSAIDs for easing arthritic pain and inflammation, and there are less of the stomach-irritating side effects associated with NSAIDs. A Chinese study of individuals with osteoarthritis of the knee found that participants taking 1,500mg of glucosamine sulphate daily had a similar reduction in symptoms to those taking 1,200mg of ibuprofen daily. However, the glucosamine group tolerated their medicine much better.[29] And in four high-quality 2005 studies of glucosamine sulphate versus NSAIDs, the glucosamine worked better in two, and was equivalent to the NSAIDs in the other two,[30] again without the side effects.

THE ROLE OF CHONDROITIN

Chondroitin, a protein that gives cartilage its elasticity, also helps the formation of proteoglycans. There is some evidence that taking glucosamine in combination with chondroitin may be even more effective in alleviating arthritis. In one such study, pain was reduced in as many as 80 per cent of volunteers who had degeneration in the knee, while inflammation was reduced in two-thirds of them.[31] The scientists reported that glucosamine appeared to produce better results overall, especially in people with mild arthritis, although chondroitin was more successful in advanced cases. Another study compared the effects of glucosamine with ibuprofen painkillers. Although the participants on the ibuprofen initially had a more dramatic reduction in pain, it stabilised after four weeks, whereas those on the glucosamine reported less pain after four and also after eight weeks.[32]

More recently, in a study funded by the US National Institutes of Health and published in 2006, researchers gave a group of 1,500 osteoarthritis patients a daily dose of either 1,500mg of glucosamine hydrochloride, 1,200mg of chondroitin sulphate, a combination of both supplements, 200mg of the prescription painkiller celecoxib (Celebrex) or a placebo. Six months later, the researchers found that both celecoxib and the glucosamine–chondroitin combination significantly reduced knee pain in those with moderate to severe pain, compared to the placebo, and better than either glucosamine or chondroitin on its own.[33]

This study, however, was widely reported as disproving the power of glucosamine because overall the supplements didn't reduce pain significantly more than the drug – or at least, only in those with higher levels of pain.[34] The abstract (the summary at the beginning) and press release failed to point out the proven benefit for those with moderate to severe pain.

Does chondroitin work as well as glucosamine?

The trouble with chondroitin is that not all supplements are of the same quality, and hence not similarly utilised by your body. And although there is evidence that chondroitin works, the research does not show that it works better than glucosamine.[35]

Most of the research has been done using glucosamine sulphate, but glucosamine hydrochloride is also known to inhibit COX-2, which means it has an anti-inflammatory effect.[36]

How much to take

Aim for 1,000 to 2,000mg of glucosamine a day (the usual dosage is 500mg, three times daily). Many people find that the longer they use it, the more beneficial it feels. It works especially well when combined with MSM (see below).

MSM FOR SULPHUR – THE BONE BUILDER

Methylsulfonylmethane, or MSM, is one of the most effective sources of the essential mineral sulphur. If you think of building cartilage as similar to building a house, glucosamine supplies the body's lengths of 'timber'. These are essential for the framework, but you also need 'nails' – and that's where sulphur comes in.

As well as glucosamine, sulphur is essential for pain relief from arthritis, because it is involved in a multitude of key body functions including pain control, inflammation, detoxification and tissue building. Some people have reported tremendous relief from arthritis by supplementing 1–3g of MSM.[37] One possible reason for this remarkable effectiveness is that sulphur deficiency is far more common than realised. A study in 1995, reported in the book *The Miracle of MSM*, found that sulphur concentration is lower in the cartilage of those with arthritis.[38] Sulphur is an essential ingredient in cartilage formation, as well as inflammatory response, and this may explain why MSM can be helpful. A number of small trials have reported consistent relief from pain and inflammation in a variety of conditions including back pain, joint pain and muscle pain.

Pain can be caused by pressure changes in cells, which in turn affect the nerves that sense pain. If cells inflate due to excess build-up of fluid or a drop in the pressure surrounding them, the nerves register the pain. Perhaps this is why people with arthritis can predict pressure changes in the weather because of the pain they experience as it is approaching. MSM may also help improve cell membrane fluidity, thereby improving the exchange of fluids in and out of cells, and reducing pressure build-up. One study at the UCLA School of Medicine found that on 2,250mg of MSM a day, patients with arthritis had an 80 per cent improvement in pain within six weeks, compared to a 20 per cent improvement in those who had taken dummy pills/placebos.[39]

A combination of both glucosamine and MSM is particularly effective.[40] An unpublished double-blind study from 2003 giving 750mg to half a group of arthritis patients and a placebo to the other half showed an 80 per cent improvement after six weeks in the first group compared to a 20 per cent improvement in the placebo group.[41]

Sulphur: how supplements can help

If you have arthritis or joint pain, I recommend that you supplement 1,000–4,000mg of glucosamine sulphate (or glucosamine hydrochloride) a day, together with 600–2,000mg of MSM. The lower end of the range is enough if you're looking to support joints and prevent their degeneration, while the higher end of the range is for those who have aching joints or a history of joint problems or arthritis, and are looking to maximise recovery. MSM is available both as a balm and in capsules. The therapeutic dose appears to be 1,500–3,000mg. It is certainly well worth trying.

Where can we find natural sources?

Foods particularly rich in sulphur include eggs, onions and garlic, but sulphur is also found in all protein foods.

RELIEF FROM THE OCEAN?

Proper controlled studies have shown benefit for both rheumatoid arthritis and osteoarthritis sufferers from supplementing green-lipped mussel extract. Although most people make enough proteoglycans (remember these, along with collagen, form cartilage), there is evidence that arthritis sufferers don't. So supplements may help.

In one study of 55 patients given green-lipped mussel extract (*Perna canaliculus*) for between six months and four and a half years, 67 per cent benefited.[42] In a double-blind study, 28 patients receiving NSAID medication were given either green-lipped mussel extract (350mg three times a day) or a placebo, for six months. Those taking the green-lipped mussel extract did significantly better than those taking the placebo.[43]

A higher proportion of rheumatoid arthritis sufferers benefit from green-lipped mussel extract. This supports other research, which suggests that proteoglycan has a significant anti-inflammatory effect as well as being a component of healthy cartilage.

How much to take

The recommended dose of green-lipped mussel extract is 1,000mg a day for 25 days, then 250mg a day. Some people experience a flare-up of symptoms within the first two weeks, before their condition improves. Obviously, this supplement is not suitable for people with an allergy to seafood.

Glucosamine v. green-lipped mussels

Overall, it is likely that glucosamine and green-lipped mussels work in much the same way. Of these two, glucosamine is the most cost-effective. Improvement is often reported after several weeks and it is therefore best to try either of these remedies for three months before judging their value for you.

BUILDING BLOCKS FOR HEALTHY JOINTS

Amino acids are the building blocks of protein, and two in particular – methionine and cysteine – may have an important role to play in restoring joint health. Methionine and its 'cousin' S-adenosyl-methionine (SAMe) are important for synthesising proteoglycans and glycoaminoglycans, which are kinds of proteoglycans, essential components of cartilage.[44] A double-blind trial, involving 150 patients, has showed SAMe to be better than NSAIDs for the treatment of osteoarthritis.[45] In another study, people with arthritis of the knee were given SAMe injections for five days, followed by SAMe tablets for three weeks, and as early as 14 days into the experiment they were in considerably less pain than a control group who were on dummy treatment.[46] Methionine is a necessary component of endorphins, the body's natural painkillers, which may also explain SAMe's pain-relieving effects. While SAMe is available over the counter in many countries, including the US and South Africa, in Europe it is classified as a medicine.

SAMe levels are generally boosted by increasing your intake of the amino acid cysteine, the precursor of glutathione, both of which are very powerful antioxidants, helping to protect joints from oxidative damage (see Chapter 10), and glutamine, which helps to detoxify and lessen the body's toxic load (see Chapter 8).

THE VITAMIN C CONNECTION

Vitamin C is vital for healthy joints. Both bone and cartilage formation depend on collagen as a building material, and collagen can be synthesised only in the presence of vitamin C. So a lack of vitamin C could quite possibly cause cartilage and bone abnormalities. The optimal intake of vitamin C is highly debatable. At the low end of the scale are government-set recommended daily amounts (RDAs), usually around 60–80mg per day. On the other hand, there is now widespread recognition that the optimal levels needed to protect against cancer and heart disease may be considerably higher than 1,000mg a day. Why the difference?

Most animals do not need to include vitamin C in their diet because their bodies produce it naturally – that is, most animals apart from guinea pigs, fruit-eating bats, the bulbul bird and primates, which includes us. So why might this be? Scientists believe that a mutation may have occurred millions of years ago that caused primates, including us, to lose the ability to produce vitamin C naturally in the body.

Mutations can and frequently do occur in nature, but only those that are advantageous to a species will tend to become dominant. Unfortunately, these are highly unlikely to be reversed. Unlike other vitamins, vitamin C is required in large amounts, and these quantities could only be supplied by a tropical diet high in fruit and other vegetation. If sufficient vitamin C could be obtained from such a diet, the quantity of glucose normally used to make it could be used for energy production instead. So, primates living in the correct conditions where they could eat plenty of vitamin C-rich foods would be at an advantage over other animals, because they would have more energy and strength.

However, this advantage may have come at a price, especially when the climate and our diet changed. Animals that don't produce vitamin C are susceptible to certain kinds of disease, particularly immune-based disease. So, could humanity's history of endemic infections, plagues and, more recently, cancer, heart disease and rheumatoid arthritis be because we can't produce vitamin C in our bodies and we don't obtain optimal amounts from the food we eat?

The fact that almost all species continue to make vitamin C suggests that the amount generally available from diet is not enough, except possibly in a tropical environment. The daily amount produced by other animals (adjusted for comparison with man) is between 3,000mg and 15,000mg – that is, an average of 5,400mg.

How much vitamin C do we need?

What about humans? Whereas a mere 60mg a day can prevent scurvy, a survey of doctors found that those who were healthiest consumed at least 250mg of vitamin C per day. A person's vitamin C status is a good predictor of their mortality risk. High vitamin C levels indicate a low risk of cardiovascular disease and certain types of cancer. Life expectancy of cancer patients has been five times higher in those given 10,000mg (10g) or more a day in oral supplements and higher amounts in intravenous drips. Optimal intakes, to reduce the risk of such conditions, may be at least 500mg a day.[47]

But aren't we simply making expensive urine when we take large amounts of supplements? Dr Michael Colgan investigated how much vitamin C we use by giving increasing daily doses and measuring excretion.[48] He concluded: 'Only a quarter of our subjects reached their vitamin C maximum at 1,500mg a day. More than half required over 2,500mg a day to reach a level where their bodies could use no more. Four subjects did not reach their maximum at 5,000mg.'

Vitamin C is not only required for the synthesis of collagen, the intercellular glue that keeps skin, lungs, arteries, digestive tract and all our organs intact. It is also a potent antioxidant, protecting us against free radicals, pollution, carcinogens, heavy metals and other toxins. It is vital for a healthy immune system and is strongly anti-viral and mildly anti-bacterial, and anti-inflammatory. It is also essential for the body's production of stress-response hormones, including natural cortisone.

How much to take

The optimum intake is likely to be anywhere between 1,000mg and 10,000mg per day. If you suffer from chronic arthritis, particularly rheumatoid arthritis, the ideal level may be in the higher range. If you drink excessive amounts of alcohol, live in a polluted city, have a stressful lifestyle, take drugs including aspirin, or smoke, your optimal intake will be raised. An intake of around 50mg per cigarette probably affords maximum protection. For anyone suffering with arthritis, 3–5g would be a sensible daily intake to assist healthy collagen formation of bone and cartilage. If you take too much you get loose bowels – a benefit for some! Many nutrition experts believe the optimal intake is the amount just below that which gives you loose bowels.

See Chapter 23 for more about supplements.

SUMMARY

In arthritic conditions where there is obvious joint degeneration and therefore cartilage depletion it may well be advisable to:

- **Supplement a cartilage rebuilder**, such as glucosamine, ideally with MSM or chondroitin, or green-lipped mussel extract, for a minimum of three months. See Chapter 23 for recommended levels.
- **Increase your intake of vitamin C** to 3–5g a day.

Although these nutrients can help reduce inflammation and rebuild cartilage, it is often more effective to deal with the underlying causes of inflammation first, as explained in Chapter 2. Maintaining bone strength is also of vital importance, as discussed in Chapter 17.

PART 4

STRATEGIES FOR OSTEOPOROSIS, FIBROMYALGIA AND GOUT

CHAPTER 17

OSTEOPOROSIS – THE SKELETON IN THE CUPBOARD

The ability to keep your bones strong depends to a large extent on how your body makes use of calcium, magnesium and phosphorus, all of which are incorporated into bone. Of these, calcium is the most abundant mineral in bone. However, more and more evidence is accumulating to show that dietary calcium intake is only one of a number of factors that influence the proper use of calcium in the body.[1] Although our calcium intake has stayed relatively constant, the incidence of osteoporosis has rocketed. Consequently, one in three women, and one in 12 men, has a fracture by the age of 70, most commonly of the hip. In the UK, 50,000 people fracture a bone as a result of osteoporosis every year – that's one every three minutes.

Yet osteoporosis is far from inevitable. In fact, in some communities, there is no apparent loss of bone density after the menopause. Even though we have a better diet, analyses of skeletal remains show less bone loss in the 18th century than the late 20th century. So what has changed? It seems to be a case of too much of some things and too little of others.

THE CALCIUM QUESTION

Unless your calcium intake is very low indeed, calcium supplementation alone makes little difference. Calcium balance in the body depends on many factors. A person with a relatively low intake of calcium, but none of the factors shown below, may have better calcium status than someone apparently consuming enough calcium, but scoring high on these factors.

Factors Influencing Bone Mass Density

Lack of	Excess of
Minerals – calcium, magnesium, boron	Protein – resulting in high levels of acidity
Vitamins – D, K, C and Bs	Refined carbohydrates – resulting in blood sugar problems
Thyroid and parathyroid hormones	
Oestrogen and progesterone – after the menopause	Stress
Exercise	Alcohol – particularly red wine
Sunlight	Stimulants – coffee, tea, cigarettes, chocolate
Stomach acid – needed to absorb minerals	Toxic elements – lead, cadmium, aluminium, fluorine

Take a look at your own diet and lifestyle over the last 20 years. Which of these factors might have contributed to the state of your bones and joints? Since most of them are the direct consequence of diet and lifestyle, which do you think is more likely to help: leaving your diet and lifestyle as it is and taking drugs; or changing your diet and lifestyle for the better? One thing is certain: there's a lot more to healthy bones than getting enough calcium.

While most of these factors have been discussed in depth earlier on in this book, two points are worth considering here. The first is the danger of too much protein; and the second is the extent to which hormone deficiencies contribute to arthritis and osteoporosis, and whether hormone replacement therapy is really advisable.

PROTEIN AND OSTEOPOROSIS

Osteoporosis is endemic in the Western world, particularly among post-menopausal women. The reason, it is thought, is that the hormone oestrogen, which ceases to be produced at the menopause, assists the retention of calcium in bone. Consequently, numerous trials have tested the effects of giving oral oestrogen, or calcium, or both. Neither have succeeded in completely 'curing' the problem, although both have an effect.

This suggests another cause, obvious when you know that many women from different cultures throughout the world have no increased incidence of osteoporosis after the menopause. Indeed, many cultural groups have no osteoporosis at all. Bantu tribes in Africa, for example, have an average calcium intake of 400mg (well below the recommended intake for post-menopausal women) and virtually no osteoporosis. In contrast, Eskimos, who consume vast amounts of calcium, have an exceptionally high incidence of osteoporosis. Why the difference? What have countries with a high incidence of osteoporosis got in common? The answer may be too much dietary protein.[2]

Although we all need something in the region of 40g (1½oz) of protein a day, eating above 80g (about 2¾oz) a day over the long term will boost your risk of developing osteoporosis. This is because protein is acidic, and excess amounts need to be neutralised, which can deplete the bones of calcium.

The Nurses' Health Study, conducted in the US and analysed by the Harvard School of Public Health, found that women who consumed 95g (3¼oz) of protein a day, as compared with those who consumed less than 68g (2¼oz) a day, had a 22 per cent greater risk of forearm fractures.[3] In another study, eating more than 80g (about 2¾oz) of protein a day, which is equivalent to bacon and eggs for breakfast and a steak for dinner, was found to increase your risk of osteoporosis.[4]

What is the link between protein and fractures?

This happens because protein is made of amino acids, and protein-rich foods therefore generate more acid in the body. Because the body cannot tolerate substantial changes in the acid pH of blood, it neutralises or 'buffers' this effect through two main alkaline agents: sodium and calcium. When the body's reserves of sodium are used up, calcium is taken from the bones – a finding that has been confirmed by metabolic 'ward' studies in which people are kept in a controlled environment, fed precise diets and measured for their calcium loss. Such studies have found that a negative calcium balance is created when 95g (3¼oz) of protein is consumed while a person eats 500mg of calcium. The calcium intake must be raised to 800mg before calcium balance is achieved – that is to say, when the calcium entering the body is the same as the amount leaving. And the more protein you eat, the more calcium you need. The difference between the Bantus and the Eskimos is their protein consumption. According to a report in the *American Journal of Epidemiology*, an 11-year study of 40,000 elderly Norwegians also found increased risk of hip fractures among those eating high amounts of non-dairy protein (meat/fish/eggs), as well as among those who had either a high coffee or low calcium intake.[5]

The fact that high-protein diets lead to calcium deficiency is nothing new. Dr Shalini Reddy from the University of Chicago conducted a six-week study on ten healthy adults eating a low-carb diet. Volunteers lost an average of 4kg (9lb) over the course of the study – that's 680g (1½lb) a week. That's the good news. The bad news was that the acid excretion in the urine, which is an indication of acid levels in the blood, rose by 90 per cent in some volunteers. There was also a sharp rise in the amount of calcium excreted in the urine during the low-carbohydrate, high-protein diets, and even the 'maintenance' diets for these regimes, despite only a slight decrease in calcium intake. This means the people were losing calcium from the body. Also, urinary citrate, a compound that inhibits kidney stone formation, decreased, implying an increased risk of kidney stone formation.[6] According to Dr Reddy, 'Consumption of a low-carbohydrate, high-protein diet for six weeks delivers a marked acid load to the kidney, increases the risk of stone formation, decreases estimated calcium balance, and may increase the risk for bone loss.' These studies all suggest that such high-protein diets may increase the risk of bone loss over the long term. Of course, we are going to have to wait a while to find out, but I'd rather you weren't the guinea pig.

The problems of a high-protein diet

Research is also beginning to show that if you eat a high-protein diet, no amount of calcium supplementation can correct the imbalance. In one study, published in the *American Journal of Clinical Nutrition*, subjects were given a moderately high protein diet (12g nitrogen) and a very high protein diet (36g nitrogen) plus 1,400mg of calcium.[7] The overall loss of calcium was 37mg per day on the moderately high diet and 137mg per day on the very high protein diet. The authors concluded that, 'high calcium diets are unlikely to prevent probable bone loss induced by high protein diets'. The negative effects of too much protein have been clearly demonstrated in patients with osteoporosis. Some medical scientists now believe that a life-long consumption of a high-protein, acid-forming diet may be a primary cause of osteoporosis.[8]

Should we eat more dairy?

Of course, the above begs the question as to whether eating a lot of dairy produce (high in both protein and calcium) would be protective or contribute to osteoporosis risk. A 12-year study which involved over 120,000 women throughout the US, found that women who drank two or more glasses of milk per day actually had a 45 per cent higher risk of hip fractures and a 5 per cent higher risk of forearm fractures than women who drank less.[9] The director of the study, Diane Feskanich, said, 'I certainly would want women to have adequate calcium in their diets, but I would not rely on that as the prime prevention against osteoporosis.' There is no clear pattern of evidence that drinking milk prevents osteoporosis.

For more information about getting the right type and amount of protein in your diet, see Chapter 21.

OSTEOPOROSIS, OESTROGEN AND HOMOCYSTEINE

As explained in Chapter 11, osteoporosis is very much linked to high blood levels of homocysteine, often a result of a lack of B vitamins. A decrease in bone mineral density resulting in osteoporosis is a common symptom of the rare genetic disease homocystinuria, which is associated with very high homocysteine levels. Research from Japan has found that women with the greatest post-menopausal bone mass loss are much more likely to have a defect in the gene MTHFR, which produces an enzyme that removes homocysteine, resulting in a higher than normal homocysteine score.[10] These women may be particularly at risk of osteoporosis unless they follow a diet and supplement plan to lower their homocysteine level.

High levels of homocysteine and fractures

A number of studies suggest that having a high level of homocysteine in your blood may weaken bone and increase the risk of fractures.[11] One of these was a very large study (involving 2,268 men and 3,070 women) by Dr Clara Gjesdal and her colleagues at the University of Bergen in Norway – known as the Hordaland Homocysteine Study – which showed that elevated homocysteine and low folate levels were associated with reduced bone mineral density in women, but not in men.[12] When it was fracture risk that was being evaluated, one study showed that risk of fracture was higher in men – almost four times higher for men; almost two times higher for women,[13] whereas another showed double the risk of fracture for both men and women.[14]

Dr Markus Hermann, from the University of Sydney, Australia, and colleagues from Germany and Italy reviewed a total of 28 studies and concluded that high homocysteine levels (and possibly B-vitamin deficiencies) have a detrimental effect on bone quality because they stimulate the cells that clear out old bone. Since there is no direct effect on the bone-*building* cells, old bone ends up being cleared away faster than new bone is produced.[15]

It is not yet clear if it is the homocysteine itself that is causing the damage to bone and increased fracture risk or whether homocysteine levels are just reflecting low levels or deficiencies of either folate or B_{12} – nutrients that *do* have a direct effect on bone.[16] Some studies suggest that low folate levels influence bone mineral density and/or fracture risk,[17] whereas others implicate B_{12}.[18] Patients with a type of anaemia, called pernicious anaemia (caused by lack of B_{12} in the blood), have decreased bone mineral density at the lumbar (lower) spine, and in comparison with the general population they have almost double the risk of hip fracture.[19]

Dr Rosalie Dhonukshe-Rutten, from Wageningen University in the Netherlands, has shown that frail elderly women with a B_{12} deficiency were seven times more likely to have osteoporosis than women with normal B_{12} levels. Older women, but not men, with low bone mineral density had significantly lower vitamin B_{12} levels than older women with higher bone mineral density.[20] This is because B_{12} has a direct effect on bone-building cells and also stimulates an enzyme involved in the process of forming new bone (called alkaline phosphatise, or ALP for short). Another of her studies showed that high homocysteine and low B_{12} were significantly associated with less bone strength, increased bone turnover and a three times higher risk of fractures in men and women. However, the impact of low B_{12} was more severe in women than men, whereas high homocysteine was more associated with fractures in men.[21]

Would supplements help?

Not many studies have been done to see what effects supplementing homocysteine-lowering nutrients have on bone mineral density and fracture risk. However, since stroke increases the risk of subsequent hip fracture by 2 to 4 times, one Japanese study followed 433 stroke patients, aged 65 and over, for 2 years to see if treatment with folate (5mg) and vitamin B_{12} (1,500mcg) would have any effect. The treatment was found to be a safe and effective way of reducing the risk of hip fracture in these patients.[22]

Low oestrogen, high homocysteine

A low level of oestrogen, which is very common in post-menopausal women, also appears to raise homocysteine and increase osteoporosis risk. Theoretically, increasing oestrogen could help lower homocysteine.[23] This has been shown in some preliminary studies,[24] but not in others. Until more is understood about how homocysteine and oestrogen are related, I am reluctant to recommend oestrogen HRT as a means to lower homocysteine for two reasons. One is that it is less effective than the nutritional strategy to lower homocysteine; the other is that it carries an increased risk of breast and uterine cancer. 'Natural' progesterone HRT (not to be confused with synthetic progestins used in most HRT preparations) does not have these associated risks (the body can convert progesterone into oestrogen if needed). But no one has yet investigated whether this lowers homocysteine.

ARE ARTHRITIS AND OSTEOPOROSIS HORMONE-DEFICIENCY DISEASES?

Hormone balance, under the control of the endocrine system, is key to bone health. The endocrine system is made up of a network of glands that secrete hormones which control many of the processes that happen inside our bodies. Hormones can be protein-like, such as insulin, or fat-like, such as cortisol. Fat-based hormones are called steroid hormones. Most hormones are themselves controlled by means of feedback. An example of this feedback mechanism is seen in the working of the pituitary gland.

Often called the 'master gland', the pituitary governs the functioning of the thyroid gland, the adrenal glands and the sex glands. The thyroid gland, in turn, controls our rate of metabolism and, together with the parathyroid glands, the balance and utilisation of calcium. The adrenal glands control our ability to deal with stress, and, together with the pancreas, the balance and utilisation of glucose (sugar). And the sex glands control the production of sex hormones, including oestrogen and progesterone (which affects how the body uses calcium). The adrenal glands also produce small amounts of sex hormones.

If you continually overuse or overstress any bodily organ or system, it will eventually under-function. If the entire endocrine system is overstressed, this can lead to slow metabolism, calcium imbalance, blood sugar imbalance, inability to cope with stress, sex hormone imbalances, and (in women)

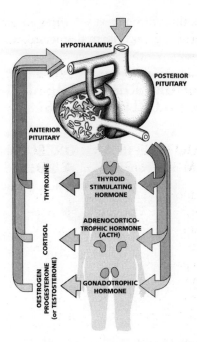

Figure 20 – The endocrine glands and hormones

premature menopause with exaggerated symptoms. I noticed that many of my arthritis patients had a history of prolonged stress, overuse of stimulants, over-consumption of refined carbohydrates, and deficiency of the many essential vitamins and minerals needed for the endocrine system to work. This prompted me to wonder whether arthritis might be caused, at least in part, by hormone imbalances created by overstressing the endocrine system as a whole. Rather than treating the effect – in other words giving hormones like cortisone, thyroxine, calcitriol and oestrogen – I experimented with treating the possible cause by encouraging my patients to change their diet and lifestyle, and to support their endocrine system by taking vitamins and minerals. This approach has proven most effective, and, although as yet unproven in clinical trials, research is beginning to confirm that it makes sense.[25]

IS OESTROGEN REALLY THE ANSWER FOR OSTEOPOROSIS?

The previous conventional treatment for osteoporosis was hormone replacement therapy (HRT), employing either oestrogen alone or a combination of oestrogen and synthetic progesterone (called progestagens in the UK and progestins in the US). There is little doubt that oestrogen therapy does increase bone density and reduce the incidence of fracture (see Figure 21, opposite). However, oestrogen HRT does also increase the risk of high blood pressure, gall bladder disease, blood clots and, most importantly, breast, uterine or endometrial cancer with or without progestagens.[26] In fact, a five-year study involving one million women aged between 50 and 64 showed that the risk is substantially greater for oestrogen–progestagen combinations than for other types of HRT.[27] Since stopping oestrogen therapy rapidly returns bone mass to its previous osteoporotic level,[28] oestrogen therapy (or other forms of HRT) is only really effective as a long-term treatment, which means a long-term risk. Consequently, few doctors continue to advise this.

The role of calcium and vitamin D

Although not so striking in effect, ensuring adequate intake of calcium, vitamin D and other nutrients, especially magnesium, does increase bone density. Vitamin D is converted into a hormone, calcitriol, which improves calcium utilisation and retention in the body. Supplementing the hormone itself may be even more effective than taking vitamin D, and, unlike oestrogen, it has no apparent significant side effects.[29]

A high calcium intake prior to the menopause does seem to improve bone density.[30] However, once osteoporosis has set in, calcium supplementation is only marginally effective in increasing bone density, except in people who eat a calcium-deficient diet.

How much to take

The recommended intake of calcium for a post-menopausal woman is in the order of 1,000–1,500mg per day. More than this is unlikely to be of any benefit.

PROGESTERONE AND BONES

Bones have two kinds of cell: osteoblasts, which build new cells; and osteoclasts, which get rid of old bone material, such as calcium. Oestrogen, which influences osteoclast cells, does not actually help build new bone. It only stops the loss of old bone. Progesterone, on the other hand, stimulates osteoblasts, which actually build new bone.[31] Taking natural progesterone increases bone density four times more than taking oestrogen (see Figure 21).

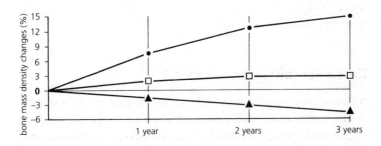

Figure 21 – The effects of natural progesterone ●, oestrogen □, or no hormone supplement ▲ on bone density

In the time leading up to the menopause, most women start to have cycles in which ovulation doesn't occur (known as anovulatory cycles). After the menopause ovulation never occurs. If no egg is released, no progesterone is produced (because progesterone is only made in the ovary sac once the egg is released). However, the body does continue to produce small amounts of oestrogen. Scientists are now starting to think that it is the relative excess of oestrogen to progesterone – creating, in effect, a progesterone deficiency – that precipitates osteoporosis, rather than the deficiency in oestrogen. This would explain why bone loss commonly starts from the age of 35, long before the actual menopause. In the pre-menopausal years, anovulatory cycles (in which no progesterone is produced) become increasingly common. Loss of bone mass density is known to occur in women who have such anovulatory cycles.[32] One trial, by Dr John Lee from California, found that giving nature-identical progesterone, as a transdermal skin cream, was four times more effective than oestrogen HRT, with none of the associated risks.[33]

NATURAL REMEDIES

Several factors in natural foods may also help to prevent osteoporosis in both men and women by keeping hormones in balance. Although too much protein (especially from red meat) causes calcium loss and encourages inflammation, switching to a lower protein intake, with a greater proportion of vegetarian protein foods, helps protect against both arthritis and osteoporosis. Most interesting is the role of a group of naturally occurring hormone-like substances called isoflavones (a type of phyto-oestrogen) found in soya. These seem to enhance bone building and prevent the breakdown of bone. Ipriflavone, a derivative of these naturally occurring isoflavones, has been extensively tested and has proven, in over a dozen trials, to increase bone density and decrease bone loss, when given with either calcium, oestrogen HRT or vitamin D, significantly more than when these are given alone.[34]

Although much attention has been focused on vitamin D and calcium, good bone health also depends on a lot of other nutrients. The minerals magnesium, zinc, manganese, boron and strontium all have a role to play in helping to build bone or cartilage. Vitamin K, antioxidants and B vitamins are also important. Women with osteoporosis often have low serum levels of vitamin K. Supplementing vitamin K decreases their loss of calcium. Therefore an all-round optimum nutrition programme, consisting of a healthy, balanced diet plus supplements containing all these nutrients, provides the best chance of keeping bones healthy.

THE EXERCISE FACTOR

One of the primary stimulants for bone growth and density is exercise, which will have profound effects on keeping your bones strong and protecting you from osteoporosis. This is because the body, unlike most mechanical devices, is unique in the way it responds to the amount of use it receives. Where most machines' components wear down with regular use, the body does the opposite by building and strengthening the areas that are being used. Stressing the bones with weight-bearing exercise tells the body to 'toughen up', which is why astronauts in zero gravity conditions rapidly lose bone density. There is little difference between them and a person who sits at work all day, drives home and sits watching television all evening. We all need some weight-bearing activity every day, such as a 30-minute walk. On top of that, more strenuous activities at least once a week – hill walking, running, cycling, exercise classes – are necessary to keep your bones strong.

Knowing this, we can start to make small changes in our lifestyle that will help to prevent the onset of osteoporosis. By making the skeleton perform load-bearing movements on a regular basis, it will respond by increasing the density of the bones being used thus making them stronger and less prone to breaks. The exercise recommendations below are for both younger individuals and women in the menopause, as prevention is vital. If you already have osteoporosis, follow the advice given for osteoporosis sufferers.

What kind of activity is best?

The two main forms of exercise that boost the health of your bones and increase bone mass are weight-bearing exercise and resistance exercise:

A weight-bearing exercise is one where bones and muscles work against the force of gravity. This is any exercise in which your feet and legs carry your weight. Examples are walking, jogging, dancing and climbing stairs.

Resistance exercise involves moving your body weight or objects to create resistance. This type of exercise uses the body areas individually, which also strengthens the bone in that particular area.

For younger individuals, including women before the menopause

You can either do all the following suggestions or a combination of them based on your level of fitness:

- Jumping or skipping on the spot (50 jumps daily).
- Jogging or walking for 30 minutes (5–7 days per week).
- Resistance weight training (2–3 days per week).
- High-impact circuit or aerobic-style class (1 or 2 times per week).

continued

For post-menopausal women and men over 50

You can either do all of the following suggestions or a combination of them based on your level of fitness:

- Weight training (one set of 8–12 repetitions using maximum effort. If 12 can be reached on a regular basis then the weight is slightly too light).
- Jogging/walking for 10–20 minutes (5–7 days per week).
- Stair climbing (10 flights of 10 steps per day).
- Exercise classes such as yoga or aqua aerobics (1 or 2 per week).

Exercise for those who have osteoporosis

People with osteoporosis should not do any of the exercises listed above. Their bones are too fragile to resist the stresses and strains, which are beneficial in stimulating bone growth in more robust individuals. However it is important that they take regular gentle exercise to maintain physical function and also to prevent further deterioration.

The following forms of exercise are recommended for people with osteoporosis:

- 10 minutes of walking daily
- Hydrotherapy and aqua aerobics
- T'ai chi

The last two are great for safely improving balance.

Whether preventing or living with osteoporosis we can definitely all benefit from regular exercise. By becoming more active in your daily life and at least taking time out to walk 10 minutes a day you should definitely feel a difference in your health within six weeks. Get pleasure from your chosen activity. If you don't like it, you won't do it! So make sure you find an activity that suits you, have fun and try something different from time to time.

THE HARD FACTS ABOUT SOFT DRINKS

Avoid artificially carbonated drinks and soft drinks containing phosphoric acid if you want to have healthy bones. Phosphoric acid is used as a preservative in many fizzy drinks. Too much means excess phosphorus, a mineral that needs to be carefully balanced with calcium. When dietary phosphorus is too high and calcium too low, the body takes calcium from the bone to handle the excess phosphorus in the blood.

Also, when you drink naturally carbonated mineral water, the carbon particles, which have a natural affinity for minerals, become bound to minerals as the water makes its way through rock to the surface spring. These carbonated minerals are taken into the body. Conversely, if you drink artificially carbonated water or drinks, it's conceivable that the carbonates might bind to minerals inside the body and take them out. But the real culprit appears to be phosphoric acid. So a regular intake of carbonated fizzy drinks with added phosphoric acid is bad news as far as bones are concerned.

WHAT YOU CAN DO TO HELP YOURSELF

In conclusion, the best advice for anyone, whether suffering from arthritis or osteoporosis, is to avoid excess protein, sugar, fizzy drinks, alcohol and stimulants and to ensure optimal intakes of vitamins and minerals including magnesium, vitamin D, boron, zinc, vitamin C and other bone-friendly nutrients. These are often provided together in one supplement. The best single food source is seeds – one heaped tablespoon of ground sesame, sunflower, flax or pumpkin seeds will give you significant amounts of calcium, magnesium and zinc, plus essential fats. Dairy produce is a good source of calcium, but a poor source of magnesium. Bear in mind that our ancestors didn't milk buffaloes; they got their calcium and other minerals from seeds, nuts and vegetables.

If hormone replacement therapy is still needed, consider natural progesterone as opposed to oestrogen HRT. The combined supplementation of vitamins and minerals, plus hormones, has not only proven more effective in restoring bone density, but is also more effective in retaining it once hormone replacement therapy is stopped.[35] Whether or not the complete approach recommended in this book – including diet, low stimulant intake, exercise and supplements – can replace hormone replacement therapy has yet to be put to the test.

The best way to prevent or reverse osteoporosis is to combine all these prevention strategies.

See Chapter 23 for more about supplements.

SUMMARY

- **Don't consume more than 40g (1½oz) of protein a day**. This is not usually a problem for vegetarians, who should aim to have two servings daily of a protein vegetable food, such as lentils, beans or tofu. For a meat-eater this means meat certainly no more than once a day and, ideally, no more than three times a week.
- **Eat fish rather than meat**. Fish is preferable, because it provides more anti-inflammatory essential fats and fewer oestrogenic hormones.
- **Rely on seeds and nuts for minerals**, not dairy products. Dairy products, especially cheese, are high in protein and oestrogenic hormones and low in magnesium. A heaped tablespoon of ground seeds gives you calcium, magnesium and many other essential nutrients.
- **Supplement a bone mineral complex**. This should include 500mg of calcium, 350mg of magnesium, 10mcg

continued

(400iu) of vitamin D, 2mg of boron, 10mg of zinc, plus vitamins C and K, and B vitamins.

- **Avoid coffee**. High coffee intake is associated with low bone density.
- **Exercise every other day**. The best kind of exercise is weight bearing, preferably using both lower and upper body muscles. Rowing, for example, is excellent. Even walking for 15 minutes each day makes a difference.
- **If appropriate, use natural progesterone cream**. If pre-menopausal, check your hormone levels and, if oestrogen-dominant, use natural progesterone. If post-menopausal, use it anyway. Your doctor can prescribe it. In case of difficulty, or for information, contact the Natural Progesterone Information Service (see Resources, page 346).

CHAPTER 18

TREATING FIBROMYALGIA, POLYMYALGIA AND MUSCLE PAIN

A growing number of people complain of moderate to severe muscle pain as they get older. As there may be no evidence of joint degeneration and inflammation, such problems are not classified as arthritis. Instead, they are often diagnosed as fibromyalgia (pain in fibrous tissue), polymyalgia (pain in many places) or fibrositis (inflammation of fibrous tissue). The differences between these can be confusing for both practitioner and patient; they are best distinguished by whether or not there is evidence of inflammation.

FIBROMYALGIA

The condition fibromyalgia (sometimes known as FM) is debilitating and frustrating, especially as it frequently goes undiagnosed, not only by doctors but also by sufferers who may feel as though they are simply run down or fighting off a bug. Chronic musculoskeletal pain is the key feature, but as any person with fibromyalgia will tell you, the pain is just the tip of the iceberg. It is often accompanied by chronic, disabling fatigue; many very tender spots on the neck, shoulders, back and hips; constant aches; general stiffness; sleep disturbances; depression; allergic rhinitis (inflammation of the mucous membrane in the nose) – and sometimes even cardiovascular problems. As such, it is similar in a number of ways to chronic fatigue syndrome, but with the addition of muscular pain.

The incidence of fibromyalgia is increasing, but clear recognition of symptoms and their cause does make effective treatment possible. Osteopaths can diagnose fibromyalgia by testing and detecting designated sensitive points on the body (see Figure 22). For reasons that are not yet understood, it appears to affect five times as many women as men. When considering a diagnosis of fibromyalgia it is very important to distinguish it from fibrositis, which is characterised by the inflammation of muscles or connective tissue.

What causes fibromyalgia?

Fibromyalgia does not arise from inflammation. Rather, research indicates that the painful muscles are caused by decreased energy production within the muscle cells themselves and the reduced ability of muscles to relax.[36] This has been linked to a deficiency in the energy molecule ATP, which is normally produced in each cell of the body to provide the fuel for its functions.[37] Without ATP, the cells (and consequently the muscle, organ or whatever tissue they are part of) cannot function optimally. In the case of fibromyalgia, the muscles fail to relax properly once they have contracted. One factor contributing to ATP deficiency is a poor oxygen supply to cells. Insufficient oxygen (called hypoxia) results in low energy production and compromised cellular function in general.

The disrupted sleep patterns experienced by many fibromyalgia sufferers can contribute further to exhaustion and anxiety. Studies carried out in France found that people diagnosed with fibromyalgia have low levels of serotonin in the brain.[38] Serotonin is a 'communication' chemical in the

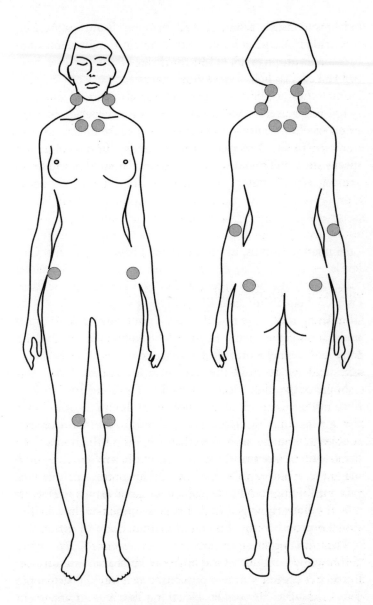

Figure 22 – Tender points in fibromyalgia

brain that is partly responsible for bringing about restful sleep. It is made from the amino acid tryptophan. Supplements of 5-hydroxytryptophan (5-HTP), in doses of 200mg one hour before bed, can help to restore restful sleep.

In studies, 5-HTP has very successfully reduced muscular symptoms as well.[39] According to Professor Federigo Sicuteri from the University of Florence, an expert in this area of research, 'In our experience, as well as in that of other pain specialists, 5-HTP can largely improve the painful picture of primary fibromyalgia.'[40]

How can it be treated?

Like many disorders, it's best to treat fibromyalgia on several levels – mechanical, chemical and emotional. So-called 'mechanical' methods of treatment (such as massage and exercise) do help to increase the supply of oxygen to tissues by stimulating the blood flow. These do not, however, address the underlying cause of the energy deficiency and pain. Indeed, some people feel worse after massage, and many feel unable to take any exercise while they are exhausted and in pain.

Some of the most successful results have come from treating fibromyalgia on a more chemical level. Research has shown that a deficiency in magnesium can lead to an increased perception of pain.[41] This in turn increases stress, which stimulates the release of stress hormones. One effect of these is to push magnesium out of cells, further depleting stores of this vital mineral.[42] This worsens muscular pain and also puts sufferers at risk of other magnesium-deficiency symptoms such as cardiovascular problems. In this way, a vicious circle of action and reaction can be set in motion.

The good news is that the cycle can be broken – researchers in the US suggest that it is possible to reverse ATP deficiency due to insufficient oxygen by taking magnesium and malic acid.[43] They report that some fibromyalgia sufferers have a significant reduction in pain after as little as 48 hours. Other nutrients that are particularly necessary for the efficient production of ATP are B vitamins, manganese and co-enzyme Q_{10}. Indeed, symptoms of a deficiency in B vitamins, particularly B_1, do resemble those of fibromyalgia. Some people with vitamin D deficiency get wrongly diagnosed with fibromyalgia.[44] Manganese is also needed for various hormonal processes that lead to thyroxine output. Thyroxine is responsible for determining metabolic rate, so any reduction in it could lead to an overall decline in metabolism and energy production.

Polymyalgia and fibrositis

Polymyalgia rheumatica (sometimes known as PMR) is another group of symptoms that respond to anti-inflammatory treatment. Classic symptoms are pain (which does not ease with rest) in many areas of the body, often in the hands, wrists, feet and arms, such that the person is unable to raise their arms above shoulder height. There is often a raised erythrocyte sedimentation rate (ESR) – a blood test that measures inflammation – and treatment frequently involves a course of steroid hormones such as prednisolone to relieve the pain. Again, this suggests a systemic problem where the body's chemistry has gone into alarm mode, indicated by the state of inflammation. The symptoms will be eased by following the advice given in Part 2.

The name fibrositis is given to diffuse, rather than acute, muscle pain that responds to anti-inflammatory treatment, be it drugs or the natural remedies recommended in Chapter 5. It is highly likely to be the cumulative effect of either digestion and detoxification problems, poor blood sugar control, too many oxidants versus antioxidants, lack of essential fats, or allergies, or a

continued

combination of such factors that eventually programme the body for inflammatory reactions. In other words, it is likely to arise from an underlying imbalance in a person's whole chemistry, so it is a case of tackling these causes rather than just suppressing the symptoms.

FIBROMYALGIA, CHRONIC FATIGUE AND HOMOCYSTEINE

A team of researchers headed by Dr Bjorn Regland at the Institute of Clinical Neuroscience at Sweden's Goteborg University ran a battery of tests on fibromyalgia sufferers, including homocysteine tests. By far the most significant finding was that every single patient with fibromyalgia had high homocysteine. They also found a direct correlation between their B_{12} status and the severity of their reported symptoms.[45] Fibromyalgia sufferers should be routinely tested for homocysteine and, if high, immediately started on a homocysteine-lowering programme (see Chapter 11). For more information on homocysteine and related conditions, read my book *The H Factor*, co-written with Dr James Braly (see Recommended Reading).

See Chapter 23 for more about supplements.

SUMMARY

The following advice may provide relief from the symptoms of fibromyalgia:

- **Eat a healthy diet**, with plenty of magnesium-rich foods such as green vegetables, nuts and seeds.
- **Supplement key vitamins and minerals** Magnesium and malic acid (magnesium malate), vitamin B complex, co-enzyme Q_{10} and a multivitamin/mineral that contains manganese.

continued

- **Supplement 5-HTP**, particularly if your symptoms include sleep problems and/or depression. The ideal dose is 100mg, three times a day, or all three tablets one hour before sleep for sleep problems. Some practitioners recommend taking 5-HTP in combination with St John's Wort (300mg three times per day, 0.3 per cent hypericin content) and magnesium (200–250mg), also three times a day.
- **Test your homocysteine level** – if it's high, follow the guidelines on page 144.
- **Reduce your stress levels** and learn how to relax. Stress-management skills can help teach relaxation. Other relaxation methods, such as yoga, t'ai chi and breathing exercises, can also be useful. Consider supplementing magnesium (300mg) as a muscle relaxant.
- **Increase exercise slowly** Exercise should be gradually increased as the fibromyalgia sufferer's capacity for it increases. Posture and overall body structure need to be optimised, perhaps with the help of an osteopath or Alexander Technique teacher. Gentle massage, heat treatment and gentle stretching also help to improve muscle function and reduce pain.
- **Also supplement**:
  - 2 × high-potency multivitamin and mineral
  - 2 × vitamin C 1,000mg
  - 2 × essential omega-3 and 6 oil capsules
  - Magnesium malate 600mg (150–250mg three times a day recommended in other sources)
  - 50–100mg 5-HTP three times a day

CHAPTER 19

....

GOODBYE TO GOUT

Gout is actually a form of arthritis, sometimes called 'gouty arthritis', and is caused by a build-up of uric acid, a substance in the blood that should be excreted from the body via the kidneys. Excess uric acid can form crystals that lodge in joints and tissue, most commonly the big toe, causing localised pain. When gout is present there is usually increased inflammation, which may affect other joints, such as ankles, heels, knees, wrists, elbows, fingers and spine.

One of the main causes is a diet containing high levels of a substance called purine, which is particularly rich in red meat and organ meat. Oily fish (such as salmon, sardines and herring) also contain purine and this can create problems in some people. Other risk factors include obesity and heavy alcohol consumption, especially beer, and particularly if there is insufficient water intake – less than 1.5 litres (2¾ pints) – per day. It normally affects middle-aged and older adults, with men being six times more likely than women to suffer from gout, although it is unlikely before the age of 30 for men and before the menopause for women.

If you are unfortunate enough to suffer from gout, you will probably be prescribed NSAIDs (in the absence of kidney or digestive problems) or another form of drug to lower urate levels. Other measures include a purine-restrictive diet, weight loss in the case of obesity and lowering alcohol intake.

SUPPLEMENT HELP FOR GOUT

Two nutrients that have shown to be effective in the treatment of gout have been mentioned previously. These are the essential fat GLA[46] and pantothenic acid, a B vitamin. The latter helps convert uric acid to urea and ammonia, which can be eliminated from the body. In the vast majority of gout sufferers, the high uric acid levels are as a result of under-excretion rather than over-production, so anything that can increase elimination from the body has to be a good thing.

A recent study in the US concluded that higher vitamin C intake is associated with a lower risk of gout and that supplementing vitamin C may help prevent it. This 20-year study, conducted by researchers from Boston University School of Medicine, involved nearly 47,000 men, of which 1,317 developed gout. Those taking 1,000–1,499mg of vitamin C per day had a 34 per cent lower risk of gout, and those who took 1,500mg or more per day had a 45 per cent lower risk. The US researchers believe vitamin C works in two ways: it eases inflammation and lowers uric acid levels in the blood.

How much to take

I believe that optimal intakes of vitamin C may be at least 500mg a day. For anyone suffering with gout, or any form of arthritis, 1.5–3g would be a sensible daily intake. As mentioned previously, if you take too much you may get loose bowels and many nutrition experts believe the optimal intake is just below that point.

THE BENEFICIAL EFFECTS OF CHERRIES AND BERRIES

Cherries, blueberries and hawthorn berries and their juice are good for gout because they contain anthocyanidins and proanthocyanidins (types of flavonoids that give these foods their deep red–blue colour). Perhaps the most exciting of these is the Montmorency tart cherry, grown in the US, which I highlighted for its exceptional antioxidant properties in Chapter 10.

As long ago as the 1950s, tart cherries have been reported to have anti-gout benefits and many people have found benefit from eating them or their juice. One study from the United States Department of Agriculture's Human Nutrition Research Center at the University of California found that consumption of cherries (two servings or 280g/10oz) after an overnight fast significantly lowered uric acid levels. There was also a decrease, although not statistically significant, in inflammation.[47] Other studies suggest that tart cherries have powerful anti-inflammatory effects, which could explain their benefit for gout sufferers.[48]

The amount usually recommended is anywhere between half a cup and one pound of cherries a day. They are either eaten or blended and then diluted with water to make a juice. Montmorency cherry extracts and concentrates are also available at some health-food stores (see Resources, page 347). Apart from being very good for you, cherry juice, made from concentrate, is a delicious daily drink.

See Chapter 23 for more about supplements.

SUMMARY

- **Take 500–1,000mg pantothenic acid** (vitamin B$_5$) each day for a trial period of two months. This may help convert uric acid to urea and ammonia and thereby speed up elimination from the body.
- **Take GLA (omega-6)** An appropriate dose is 200–300mg per day, reducing to 150mg after three months, if inflammation lessens and symptoms remain stable. Since evening

continued

primrose oil (EPO) contains about 10 per cent GLA, this means supplementing 2,000–3,000mg (usually 4–6 500mg capsules) of EPO initially, reducing to 1,500mg (3 500mg capsules).

- **Take 1.5–3g of vitamin C** Start with 1g and then build up until you get loose bowels (the optimal intake is the amount just below that which gives you loose bowels).
- **Take Montmorency cherry extracts** and concentrates as a daily drink or eat between half a cup and 450g (1lb) of tart cherries a day, if suffering from a gout attack.
- **Consume other red–blue berries**, such as blueberries, regularly as part of a prevention strategy.

PART 5

REVERSE ARTHRITIS NOW

CHAPTER 20

THE MYTH OF THE WELL-BALANCED DIET

At the Institute for Optimum Nutrition we advise people with a range of health problems, including arthritis and osteoporosis, and have found that improvements in health are linked to specific changes in the diet as well as supplementing with vitamins and minerals. Although we all know that it's important to eat a balanced diet, the greatest lie in healthcare today is that 'as long as you eat a well-balanced diet you get all the nutrients you need'. This is a lie because no single piece of research in the last few decades has managed to show that people who consider themselves to be eating a well-balanced diet are actually receiving all the recommended daily amounts (RDAs) of vitamins and minerals, let alone those levels of nutrients that are consistent with optimum nutrition.

WHAT IS A WELL-BALANCED DIET?

When conventional nutritionists are asked what a well-balanced diet is, they define it as a diet that provides all the nutrients you need; but it's not always possible to do this, or to even know that the food you eat actually has those nutrients contained within it. It's a Catch-22 situation. According to Dr Stephen Davies, Medical Director of London's Biolab Medical

Unit, 'these people are nutritional flat-earthers because they employ a thought process akin to that which was adopted by the original flat-earthers, those who maintained that the world was flat, rather than round, despite overwhelming evidence to the contrary'.[1]

The reality is that the vast majority of us are deficient in a number of essential nutrients, including vitamins, minerals, essential fats and amino acids (the constituents of protein). Deficient means 'not efficient' – in other words, we are not functioning as efficiently as we could because we have an inadequate intake of one or more nutrients. If this comes as a shock, consider the following six facts:

1 **RDAs are not optimum**. According to the National Academy of Sciences, who set US RDAs, 'RDAs are neither minimal requirements nor necessarily optimal levels of intake'. Factors considered to raise one's requirements considerably above RDA levels include alcohol consumption, smoking, exercise habits, pregnancy, times of stress (including puberty and premenstrual phases), pollution, special dietary habits (such as vegetarianism), and chronic illness such as arthritis.
2 **RDAs vary from country to country**. A five-fold variation from one country to another is not at all uncommon.
3 **RDAs don't exist for many essential nutrients**. There are 45 known essential nutrients. In Europe RDAs exist for fewer than half of these.
4 **The majority of people do not achieve RDA levels from their diet**. A government survey in 1990 showed that the average person does not get the RDA for iron.[2] An independent survey in 1985 found that over 90 per cent of people consumed less than the US RDA for vitamin B_6 and folic acid.[3] A government report stated that 10 per cent of the British population consume less than 30mg of vitamin C.[4] The RDA is 60mg. More than a third of people over 60 years old are B_{12} deficient.[5]

5 **Food does not contain what you think it contains**. Most of
these surveys are based on recording what people eat and
looking up what those foods contain in standard textbooks.
But do they take into account the fact that an orange can
contain anything from 180mg of vitamin C to none?[6] Like-
wise, a 100g (3½oz) serving of spinach can contain 158mg of
iron or as little as 0.1mg, depending on where it was grown.
Wheatgerm can contain anywhere from 21iu of vitamin E to
3.2iu. Carrots – that reliable source of vitamin A – can provide a massive 18,500iu or a mere 70iu. Organic food has
been shown to have a higher nutrient content. Store an
orange for two weeks and its vitamin C content will be
halved. Boil a vegetable for 20 minutes and 50 per cent of its
B vitamins will be gone.[7] Refine brown flour to make white
and 78 per cent of the zinc, chromium and manganese are
lost.[8] So, as you can see, it is not always possible to rely on
these standard textbook figures. The vitamin and mineral
content of the foods we eat today can vary greatly depending
on where it was grown, how long it has been stored, how it
has been cooked and so on.

Variations in nutrient content in common foods

Nutrient	Variation (per 100g of food)
Vitamin A in carrots	70–18,500iu
Vitamin B$_5$ in wholewheat flour	0.3–3.3mg
Vitamin C in oranges	0–116mg
Vitamin E in wheatgerm	3.2–21iu
Iron in spinach	0.1–158mg
Manganese in lettuce	0.1–16.9mg

6 **There is a sliding scale of deficiency**. Even if we all ate the
RDA levels, some people would still show signs of deficiency. For the vast majority these would not be the severe
symptoms of scurvy, beriberi or pellagra, but they might

well show symptoms such as skin problems, lethargy, poor concentration, frequent infections, allergies and joint aches.

MORE PEOPLE ARE MALNOURISHED THAN YOU MAY REALISE

The sad truth is that more suffering is caused by malnutrition, both in the West and in less developed countries, than by any other cause. According to the US Surgeon General, of the 2.1 million people in the US who die each year, 1.5 million (or 68 per cent) die from diet-related diseases. In Britain, three-quarters of people die from cardiovascular disease, cancer and complications of diabetes, all of which are clearly associated with dietary excesses, deficiencies or environmental factors. At the Institute for Optimum Nutrition, advice is given to people with a wide range of problems including digestive disorders, skin problems, cardiovascular disease, cancer, infections, headaches, hormonal problems and diabetes, as well as arthritis. The percentage of clients who improve, according to client assessment, is 86 per cent.[9]

There is no question that most people are sub-optimally nourished and unlikely to achieve an ideal intake of all nutrients from their diet alone. Changing your diet in specific ways as well as taking additional supplements is probably the most important way to both prevent and reverse arthritis and osteoporosis.

Boost your diet

To get all the nutrients you need for overall good health and to fight arthritis, you should:

- **Take a high potency multivitamin/mineral** every day.
- **Eat food as quickly as possible** after buying it.

continued

- **Eat vegetables raw** or very lightly cooked.
- **Choose wholegrains and wholefoods**, rather than refined foods.
- **Buy organic produce** whenever possible.

CHAPTER 21

THE ANTI-ARTHRITIS DIET

The best kind of diet to combat arthritis is one that is high in vitamins and minerals, with sufficient but not excessive protein. It also needs to be high in slow-releasing, low-GL carbohydrate foods and low in fast-releasing sugar, low in overall fat but with a high proportion of essential fats, and low in stimulants and alcohol. Certain foods have been noted as being particularly beneficial for arthritis. Others may be better avoided, such as foods with a high allergenic potential, especially if allergy testing has confirmed that you do react to them. The anti-arthritis diet recommended in this book is intended to reduce your overall toxic and allergic load by decreasing foods that either irritate the digestive tract, interfere with detoxification or have a high allergic potential.

One of the big problems with describing an anti-arthritis diet, however, is that each one of us is unique. No two people react to the same foods. Although this diet represents the best 'middle ground', you are more likely to maximise your health by seeing a nutritional therapist who can design a diet especially for you.

This chapter will clarify the misunderstandings many people have regarding how much protein they need to eat to be healthy. I also explain the benefits of a vegetable-based diet and how much you should aim to eat of different foods, as well

as which foods you should avoid. You will also find menus for
the first 14 days of your anti-arthritis diet, to be used in conjunction with the recipes in the next chapter.

PROTEIN MYTHS

Which words do you associate with protein? Meat, eggs and
cheese; muscles and growth; you need to eat those foods to
grow big and strong; that protein in meat is more usable than
the protein in plants; that if you do muscle-building exercise
you need more protein? Right or wrong? Many myths about
protein abound, including which are the best food sources and
how much you need to eat.

What exactly is protein?

The word protein is derived from *protos* (a Greek word meaning 'first'), because protein is the basic material of all living
cells. The human body is, for example, made up of approximately 65 per cent water and 25 per cent protein. Protein is
made out of nitrogen-containing molecules called amino
acids. Some 25 types of amino acid are pieced together in
varying combinations to make different kinds of protein,
which form the material for our cells and organs in much the
same way that letters make words that combine to form sen-
tences and paragraphs.

There are eight basic amino acids, and most of the remaining 17 can be made from them. These eight are termed 'essential amino acids' and the body cannot function without them,
although others are semi-essential under certain conditions.

Each one deserves its own optimal daily amount, although
these have yet to be set in government guidelines. The balance
of these eight amino acids in the protein of any given food
determines its quality or usability. So, how much protein do
you need and what is the best-quality?

ARE YOU GETTING ENOUGH PROTEIN?

Estimates for protein requirement vary depending on who you speak to. This is not so surprising as we are all born biochemically unique. In some countries the estimate is as low as 2.5 per cent of total calorie intake. The World Health Organization builds in a safety margin and recommends around 10 per cent of total calories from protein, or about 35g (1¼oz) of protein a day. Human breast milk, sufficient for the rapid growth of infants, derives 5 per cent of its calories from protein. The World Health Organization suggests that an infant needs relatively twice as much protein as an adult, so it is certainly unlikely that an adult would require more than 5 per cent of total calories from protein. This equates to, at most, 20g (a bit less than 1oz) of protein for the average adult male. The estimated average requirement per day, according to the Department of Health, is 36g (1¼oz) for women and 44g (1½oz) for men. If the quality of protein eaten is high, less needs to be eaten. The chart on page 237 shows a variety of foods and how much you would need to eat to obtain 20g of protein.

Good protein sources

So, which foods provide more than 10 per cent of calories from protein? You may be surprised to learn that virtually every single lentil, bean, nut, seed, grain and most vegetables and fruit provide more than 10 per cent protein. In soya beans 54 per cent of the calories come from protein, compared with 26 per cent in kidney beans. Grains vary from 16 per cent for quinoa to 4 per cent for corn. Nuts and seeds range from 21 per cent for pumpkin seeds to 12 per cent for cashew nuts. Fruit goes from 16 per cent for lemons to 1 per cent for apples. Vegetables vary from 49 per cent for spinach to 11 per cent for potatoes.

What this means is that if you are eating enough calories you are almost certainly getting enough protein, unless you are living off high-sugar, high-fat junk food. This may come as a surprise, contradicting all we are taught about protein. Yet the fact of the matter is it is difficult to obtain a mixed vegetable diet which will produce an appreciable loss of body protein.

But isn't animal protein better quality than plant protein?

ANIMAL OR VEGETABLE?

Once again, there are a few surprises when we compare the protein from animal or vegetable sources. Top of the class is quinoa (pronounced 'keenwa'), a high-protein grain from South America that was a staple food of the Incas and Aztecs. Soya too does well. Most vegetables are relatively low in the amino acids methionine and lysine; however, beans and lentils are rich in methionine. Soya beans and quinoa are excellent sources of both lysine and methionine. However, the body needs all the eight essential amino acids that makes these foods more 'complete' protein, and hence more usable by the body. Vegetarians are less prone to osteoporosis than meat eaters[10] and lose less calcium from their bones than meat eaters between the critical ages of 30 and 60.[11]

Early theories, such as those first expounded by Frances Moore Lappe in her groundbreaking vegetarian cookbook *Diet for a Small Planet*, suggested that vegetable proteins had to be carefully combined with complementary proteins to match the quality given by animal proteins. However, we have since learned that careful combining of plant-based proteins is quite unnecessary. As Frances Moore Lappe says in her revised book, 'With a healthy, varied diet, concern about protein complementarity is not necessary for most of us.'

Even so, you can increase the effective quality of the protein you eat by combining foods from different groups so that low levels of certain amino acids in one food group are made up

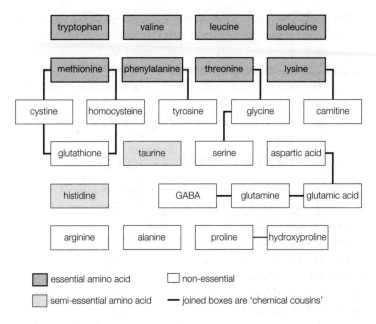

Figure 23 – The amino acid family

For a protein food source to contain 'complete' protein it must contain the eight essential amino acids. This is what you find in meat, fish, eggs, soya and quinoa. The semi-essential amino acids are also found in these foods. Taurine appears to be essential in infancy.

by high levels in another. Over a 48-hour period, aim to eat a varied diet across the food groups shown in Figure 24 overleaf. The combination of rice with lentils, for example, increases the protein value by a third. This is, of course, the basis of the diet in the Indian subcontinent.

HOW MUCH SHOULD YOU EAT?

I recommend you eat a serving of lean meat a maximum of four times a week, eat fish a minimum of three times a week,

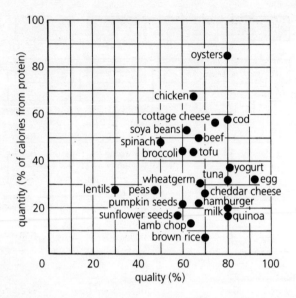

Figure 24 – Quality and quantity of protein in foods

and if you're not allergic or intolerant, have a serving of a soya-based food (tofu, tempeh, soya sausages, etc.) or beans such as kidney beans, hummus (made from chickpeas) or baked beans, at least five times a week.

What you are aiming for is two servings of protein a day, with at least one from a vegetable source and the other from a vegetable or animal source, emphasising fish and free-range or organic eggs. The chart opposite gives you the serving size of different sources of protein, each giving you 20g (¾oz) of protein. Assuming you are not a competitive or endurance athlete (who needs more high-quality protein), you need, on average, two to three of these servings, that is, 40–60g (1½–2⅛oz) of protein a day.

Protein quantities of different foods

Food	Percentage of calories as protein	Quantity of food needed to provide 20g (¾oz) protein	Protein quality
Grains/pulses			
Quinoa	16	100g (3½oz)/1 cup dry weight	Excellent
Tofu	40	275g (9¾oz)/1 packet	Reasonable
Corn	4	500g (1lb 2oz)/3 cups cooked weight	Reasonable
Brown rice	5	400g (14oz)/3 cups cooked weight	Excellent
Chickpeas	22	115g (4oz)/ ⅔ cup cooked weight	Reasonable
Lentils	28	85g (3oz)/1 cup cooked weight	Reasonable
Fish/meat			
Tuna, canned	61	85g (3oz)/1 small can	Excellent
Cod	60	35g (1oz)/1 very small piece	Excellent
Salmon	50	100g (3oz)/1 very small piece	Excellent
Sardines	49	100g (3oz)/1 baked	Excellent
Chicken	63	75g (2¾oz)/1 small roasted breast	Excellent
Nuts/seeds			
Sunflower seeds	15	185g (6oz)/1 cup	Reasonable
Pumpkin seeds	21	75g (2¾oz)/ ½ cup	Reasonable
Cashew nuts	12	115g (4oz)/1 cup	Reasonable
Almonds	13	115g (4oz)/1 cup	Reasonable
Eggs/dairy			
Eggs	34	115g (4oz)/2 medium	Excellent
Yogurt, natural	22	450g (1lb)/3 small pots	Excellent
Cottage cheese	49	125g (4oz)/1 small pot	Excellent
Vegetables			
Peas, frozen	26	250g (9oz)/2 cups	Reasonable
Other beans	20	200g (7oz)/2 cups	Reasonable
Broccoli	50	40g (1oz)/ ½ cup	Reasonable
Spinach	49	40g (1oz)/ ⅔ cup	Reasonable

continued

Food	Percentage of calories as protein	Quantity of food needed to provide 20g (¾oz) protein	Protein quality
Combinations			
Lentils and rice	18	125g (4oz)/1 small cup dry weight	Excellent
Beans and rice	15	125g (4oz)/1 small cup dry weight	Excellent

Milk – who needs it?

Not only is it possible to have a healthy diet without including dairy produce, but excessive dairy-product consumption is almost certainly contributing to a number of epidemic Western diseases. My general advice for everyone is to cut down on dairy produce. The arguments usually advanced in favour of dairy produce are its protein, calcium and vitamin content. There are, however, many excellent alternative sources of protein. As for calcium, dairy produce may not be the best source after all. Good sources of calcium include nuts (almonds, Brazil nuts), seeds (sesame, sunflower, pumpkin), pulses (soya flour, tofu, haricot beans), vegetables (spinach, cabbage, kale, carrots), and fruits (apricots, figs, rhubarb). Regarding vitamins, good sources of vitamin D are fatty fish such as herring, mackerel, pilchards, sardines and tuna, as well as eggs. There's a little in milk, meat and fortified foods. But, with sufficient exposure to sunlight, enough vitamin D may be made in the skin. Nevertheless, to be on the safe side, it is wise to take a multivitamin containing 10mcg (400iu) of vitamin D if your diet contains little meat, fish, eggs or milk. Many foods designed for vegans, such as soya milk, also contain added vitamin D.

continued

A comparison of human milk with cow's or goat's milk reveals some interesting facts. Firstly, human milk has three times as much protein, as well as substantially more calcium. Secondly, cow's milk has a higher phosphorus-to-calcium ratio; and animal studies have shown that a relatively high intake of phosphorus to calcium induces osteoporosis. Calcium and phosphorus have a complicated relationship: they are bound together in bone. When calcium is released into the blood, phosphorus is too, only to be excreted via the kidneys. A high dietary phosphorus intake may therefore mean that less 'free' calcium is available to counteract over-acidic blood, effectively inducing calcium deficiency.

Significantly, the UK, which represents 20 per cent of the EU population, consumes 40 per cent of the region's dairy produce. And our current excessive consumption of dairy produce certainly does not seem to be helping to prevent osteoporosis. Also, as I explained in Chapter 17, excessive protein consumption is a risk factor for developing osteoporosis, so it seems that increasing dairy products – a major source of protein in the average diet – is by no means the best way of ensuring adequate calcium intake.

THE FATS OF LIFE

Two people with rheumatoid arthritis obtained relief within days, which lasted for nine and 14 months respectively, by going on a low-fat diet. Within 48 hours of returning to a high-fat diet they experienced their old symptoms again.[12] These observations have been reported by other rheumatoid arthritis sufferers and suggest that the effect of a low-fat diet is far more than simple weight reduction (which could be expected to reduce arthritic symptoms in the long term, not within 48 hours). One possible explanation could be that diets containing saturated fat block the conversion of essential fats into anti-inflammatory prostaglandins. By removing all fat, anti-inflammatory prostaglandin activity may be improved.

Although I recommend a low-fat diet, I do not recommend a no-fat diet. In view of the importance of essential fats found in fish, nuts, seeds and their oils, the ideal anti-arthritis diet should be very low in saturated fat, and sufficient in these essential fats. In practical terms this means eating more vegetarian foods, since most of our saturated fat comes from meat, eggs and dairy produce.

A vegan diet (which excludes meat, fish, eggs and dairy produce) has many benefits, and is a guaranteed way to reduce saturated fat. However, it runs the risk of vitamin D and B_{12} deficiency, so these vitamins must be supplemented by vegans. Also, vegan sources of omega-3 (flax seeds) aren't nearly as potent as marine sources (fish oils), so this is another potential area where a strict vegan diet is compromised. As long as seeds and nuts, or their oils, are included, a vegan diet should encourage the body to produce anti-inflammatory prostaglandins. In one clinical study 20 rheumatoid arthritis sufferers went on a vegan diet, which also excluded coffee, tea, sugar, alcohol, salt and spices. After four months, 12 reported feeling better, five reported no change and three felt worse. Most felt less pain and were better able to function, although objective measures of grip strength didn't change.[13] (Of course, it is always hard to know whether these patients would have been expected to get worse over four months anyway.)

BENEFICIAL FOODS

The vast majority of the vitamins and minerals we need come from vegetables and fruit, so these food groups should make up 50 per cent of the food we eat. This means eating three pieces of fruit a day and large amounts of vegetables with meals. Most vegetables are best eaten raw, or lightly cooked (steaming is best).

Anti-inflammatory foods

As mentioned in Chapter 19, cherries, blueberries and hawthorn berries and their juice are good for gout because they contain anthocyanidins and proanthocyanidins (types of flavonoids that give these foods their deep red-blue colour). They have also been shown to help enhance collagen strength and to have anti-inflammatory effects.[14] Quercetin, discussed in Chapter 5 and found in onions, broccoli, squash and red grapes, is another example of a naturally occurring flavonoid with good anti-inflammatory properties.

Foods with sulphur-containing nutrients

Onions and garlic are rich in the sulphur-containing amino acids cysteine and methionine. These amino acids are essential constituents in both cartilage and antioxidant enzymes. There is some evidence that sulphur itself may benefit arthritis.[15] (Most hot springs contain water rich in sulphur, which can be absorbed into the body, and this is one reason for the reputed benefits of these remedial baths.[16])

Eggs are also a rich source of protein, especially sulphur-containing amino acids, and an excellent source of brain-boosting phospholipids. In case you didn't know, they don't raise your cholesterol level. I recommend six a week. Some people are allergic to them, however, as explained in Chapter 9. The kind of fat in an egg depends very much on the feed the chicken has been given. If the feed is rich in essential fats, then so is the egg. So it is best to eat genuinely free-range eggs, boiled rather than fried to minimise free radicals.

Foods for detoxifying

Kale, cauliflower, broccoli, cabbage and Brussels sprouts are all rich in glucosinolates, which improve detoxification capacity and thus help prevent inflammation.

Best anti-inflammatory foods

Other foods well known for their anti-inflammatory effects are:

Berries	Red onion
Flax seeds	Mackerel
Omega-3-rich eggs	Pumpkin seeds
Garlic	Salmon
Herring or kippers	Sardines
Olives	Turmeric
Red grapes	

Omega-3 and 6-rich seeds

Seeds and nuts are an important source of vitamins, minerals and essential fats. The best way to obtain the perfect balance of omega-3 and omega-6 fats, plus a generous amount of calcium, magnesium and other minerals, is to have a tablespoon of ground seeds on your morning breakfast. It is best to have half flax seeds and half others (sesame, sunflower and pumpkin) and store them un-ground in a sealed glass container in the fridge. (The reduced light, heat and oxygen exposure helps preserve the essential fats.) Then, in the morning, put a handful in your now-redundant coffee grinder and grind them up to maximise the digestion and absorption of nutrients (see Essential Seeds for Essential Health, pages 248–9).

Healthy fish and meats

Fish is another important source of essential fats and is a healthy alternative to meat. If you do eat meat, however, the best choice is probably wild game (rather than farmed meat) because it has less saturated fat and no antibiotics. Organic meat is also a good alternative. Choose free range, preferably organic chicken and don't eat the skin.

Health and flavour from herbs and spices

Use plenty of herbs and spices. Turmeric is especially beneficial and so are black pepper, cinnamon, cumin, dill, ginger,
oregano, parsley, rosemary, tarragon and thyme. However, chilli
pepper, cayenne pepper and paprika don't suit everyone. As
described in Chapter 9, it's a case of excluding them from your
diet and seeing if it makes any difference to your symptoms.

THE ANTI-ARTHRITIS 14-DAY ACTION PLAN

What you eat every day is probably the single most important
factor in protecting yourself from arthritis, over which you
have direct control. You can find out just how important diet
is for you by following this simple, 14-day diet, designed to
reverse the factors that often contribute to arthritis and related
conditions. The anti-arthritis diet:

- Provides optimum nutrition – the nutrients you need to stay
  healthy.
- Includes foods that reduce inflammation and help rebuild
  cartilage and bone.
- Excludes foods that add to the body's toxic burden.
- Excludes foods that have a high allergy potential.

Many of the foods and drinks we consume contain toxins or
trigger allergic reactions. By following this diet strictly for two
weeks, together with taking appropriate supplements, you can
break the vicious circle of disease, allowing the digestive tract
to heal, the body to detoxify and to stop reacting allergically,
and for inflammation to calm down.

It is quite possible that you may feel worse during the first
three days of this diet. This happens for a small minority of
people and is usually a sign that your body is detoxifying.
Alternatively, it might be the effects of withdrawal from either
a stimulant or an allergy-provoking food that you have
become 'addicted' to. Symptoms may include headaches,

aching muscles and joints, tiredness or slight nausea. By the third day, however, most people feel physically fitter and mentally sharper. If the symptoms do persist for more than three days, and there is no sign of improvement, seek the advice of a nutritional therapist (see Resources, page 344).

Keeping track of progress

Instead of monitoring your symptoms every week, use the system described in Chapter 26 to monitor your symptoms every day. If you notice a definite improvement in any of your symptoms over the 14 days, use this opportunity to identify whether you are allergic or intolerant to any of the foods you've been avoiding. This you can do by using the Pulse Test explained in Chapter 9, as you reintroduce certain foods one by one.

After 14 days, a number of the foods listed here can be reintroduced (see Chapter 9) while checking to see if they are causing you any ill effects.

Eat what's good; avoid what's not so good

Here are the guidelines for the first 14 days:

Foods to include and exclude

Food Group	Include	Exclude
Fruits	Fresh, frozen or canned (unsweetened) fruits, fruit juices (except those specifically prohibited)	All citrus fruits: oranges, grapefruit, lemons, limes
Grains	Non-gluten grains – brown rice, millet, buckwheat, quinoa, amaranth, tapioca	Gluten grains: wheat, corn, oats, barley, spelt, kamut, rye

continued

Food Group	Include	Exclude
Breads/cereals	Any breads/cereals made from rice, buckwheat, millet, soya, tapioca, arrowroot, amaranth, quinoa, pasta, rice noodles, rice cereal, millet flakes, rice cakes	All wheat, oats, spelt, kamut, rye, barley or gluten-containing breads and cereals
Meat/fish/eggs	All fresh fish such as halibut, salmon, cod, sole, trout; wild game, chicken, turkey, lamb	Beef, pork, cold cuts, frankfurters, sausage, canned or processed meats, eggs, shellfish
Legumes/nuts/seeds	Beans, peas, lentils; almonds, cashew nuts, walnuts, sesame (tahini), sunflower, pumpkin, and nut butters made from these	Peanuts, pistachio nuts, peanut butter
Dairy products	Milk substitutes such as rice milk, soya milk, nut milk, cashew cream (made by blending cashew nuts with water)	Milk, cheese, cottage cheese, cream, yogurt, butter, ice cream, frozen yogurt, non-dairy creamers
Vegetables	Raw, steamed, sautéed, juiced or baked vegetables (except those prohibited)	All nightshade family vegetables: tomatoes, all potatoes (except yams and sweet potatoes), aubergines and red, green and yellow peppers
Fats	Cold-pressed olive, flax seed, canola, safflower, sunflower, sesame, walnut, pumpkin, almond oils; dressings made from these oils; tahini	Margarine, butter, shortening, processed oils, salad dressing not made with included oils, spreads
Drinks	Filtered or distilled water every day, herbal tea, rooibosch (red bush tea), fruit teas	Sweetened fizzy drinks, alcoholic beverages, coffee, tea, all caffeinated beverages
Spices	Cinnamon, cumin, dill, garlic, ginger, oregano, parsley, rosemary, tarragon, thyme, turmeric	Cayenne pepper, paprika, chilli

continued

Food Group	Include	Exclude
Sweets and sweeteners	Xylitol, agave syrup, dried fruit bars (date free), fresh fruit, small quantities of dried fruit	White or brown sugar, honey, maple syrup, corn syrup, high fructose corn syrup, chocolate bars and other confectionery

Most of all, fill yourself up with lots of fruit and vegetables, rice, beans, lentils, tofu, fish and gluten-free grains. Half the world lives off these foods alone, so you should manage to do it for 14 days! Buy the freshest ingredients, organic if possible, as these tend to contain more nutrients. You'll find lots of delicious and simple recipes that follow these guidelines in my book *The Optimum Nutrition Cookbook*, co-authored with Judy Ridgway, as well as *Food GLorious Food* and *The Holford Low-GL Diet Cookbook*, co-authored with Fiona McDonald Joyce.

Drinks

It is important to drink plenty of water while you are on this diet. Aim for six to eight glasses, or 1.5 litres (2¾ pints) a day (as pure water or herb/fruit teas). If your body is eliminating toxic materials, drinking water will dilute them, thereby giving the kidneys, which cleanse the blood, an easier task. Instead of tea and coffee, choose from the wide variety of tasty alternatives available in any health-food store. Spicy teas and ginger teas are especially good for their anti-inflammatory effect. If you are a tea addict, drink rooibosch (red bush) tea instead, with some soya or rice milk. This is a staple caffeine-free drink in South Africa and is the closest thing to regular tea. You can also make your own teas. For example, try fresh ginger and cinnamon: put six large slices of ginger and a stick of cinnamon in a vacuum flask half-full of boiling water and leave to infuse for 15 minutes before you drink it.

continued

Pure apple or orange juice is fine as long as it is sugar-free and you dilute it 50 per cent with water to reduce the overall sweetness. Cherry juice, made from concentrate, is particularly beneficial (see Chapters 10 and 19). When watermelon is in season, you can make a delicious drink by blending the entire flesh, pips and all. The husks of the seeds crack and sink to the bottom leaving the white seed, full of nutrients, in the drink. A 1.2 litre (2 pint) serving is a meal in itself and thoroughly detoxifying. Vegetable juice is also excellent. Two-thirds carrot juice and one-third beetroot juice is my favourite. Carrot and apple juice is another good combination, although you may need to dilute this a little, as it is quite sweet.

THE BENEFITS OF SUPPLEMENTS

As well as following this diet, you need to take supplements, including vitamins, minerals, essential fats and anti-inflammatory herbal remedies, as explained throughout the book. Two vitamins that specifically help to speed up detoxification of the body are B_3 in the form of niacin and vitamin C. Niacin is different from niacinamide, which was recommended earlier for increasing joint flexibility. The niacin form of vitamin B_3 is a 'vasodilator', which means that it dilates or enlarges the tiny blood vessels called capillaries that deliver nutrients to cells and collect toxins. This helps them to nourish and detoxify cells.

Niacin consequently causes a temporary 'blush'. Your body goes red, a bit like mild sunburn, and you may get hot and a little itchy. This usually takes up to 15 minutes to happen, lasts for up to 30 minutes and is neither harmful nor unusual. In fact, it is very beneficial and illustrates just how potent nutrients are. Experiment with taking 100mg each day on an empty stomach. (Make sure you buy niacin, not niacinamide.)

As you can get a little cold after a niacin blush, this is a great time to have a hot bath. It's best to take niacin in the evening, in the comfort of your own home – not at work or in a potentially stressful environment. Initially your joints may ache more during the blush, and then show improvement. The after-effects of niacin are very calming and may also help to give you a good night's sleep.

Vitamin C also helps the body to detoxify, so I recommend taking 3g (three 1,000mg tablets, one with each meal) each day during these 14 days, in addition to your supplement programme (see Chapter 23).

TAKE IT EASY

During the two weeks of your diet, do your best to take it easy. Make sure you get enough sleep. Do not overstress, overwork or over-exercise yourself (although a moderate amount of exercise is still advisable). Stock up with the foods, drinks and supplements you need in advance. Any health-food store will have most of the specialist foods and drinks mentioned here.

To help you get started, I've provided ideas for healthy breakfasts, main meals, salads and desserts. The recipes are given in the next chapter and almost all are sugar-free, using the natural sweetness present in food. They are also high in fibre, so you don't need to add any. The foods used are naturally high in vitamins and minerals. For snacks, choose fruit, as many are best digested on their own; or have them with a few almonds or sunflower seeds.

Seeds are a great source of minerals, especially calcium and magnesium. As you are on a dairy-free diet, I recommend having a heaped tablespoon of ground seeds (see page 249) every day, on your morning cereal.

Essential seeds for essential health

Smart animals – from parrots to people – eat seeds. Seeds are incredibly rich in essential fats, minerals, vitamin E, protein and fibre. You need a tablespoon a day for 100 per cent health. Here's the magic formula:

1   Half-fill a glass jar that has a sealing lid with flax seeds (also known as linseeds, and rich in omega-3) and half with a mixture of sesame, sunflower and pumpkin seeds (rich in omega-6).
2   Keep the jar sealed and in the fridge to minimise damage from light, heat and oxygen.

Put a handful in a coffee or nut grinder, grind up and put a tablespoon on your cereal. Store the remainder in the fridge and use over the next few days.

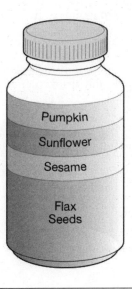

Steam-frying – the healthy alternative

A few recipes refer to 'steam-frying'. This is quite different from frying and doesn't generate harmful oxidants.
Use a tiny smear of butter or olive oil, just to lightly coat
the pan. Warm the oil and add the ingredients. As soon as
they are sizzling, add 2 tablespoons of water or vegetable
stock and cook with the lid on. In this way vegetables
can be 'steam-fried', using a fraction of the fat used in
frying, and still taste delicious. Some lunches and dinners
give quantities for two or four people. So don't forget to
divide the quantities accordingly if you're just cooking
for yourself.

MENUS – THE FIRST 14 DAYS

Here is a list of suggested menus to help you (recipes are given
in the next chapter). Any of these meals can be swapped by
others in the menus. The key points are to stay off the foods
and drinks in the 'exclude' column on pages 244–6, eat plenty
of fruit and vegetables and drink plenty of water. For mid-
morning or mid-afternoon snacks, you can have a piece of
fruit, plus five almonds or two teaspoons of pumpkin seeds.
Choose from apples, pears, plums, cherries, berries and
peaches. You can eat an entire punnet, or even more, of berries
such as strawberries, cherries and blueberries, but if you are
trying to lose weight, avoid bananas; although they're fine with
Get Up & Go for breakfast, they have too high a GL (a 120g
(4¼oz) banana is 12 GLs) to have as an additional snack.

Days 1, 6 and 11

BREAKFAST
Get Up & Go

LUNCH
Beany Vegetable Soup and Green Salad

DINNER
Chicken with Roasted Courgettes and Red Onion
Fruit Juice Jelly

Days 2, 7 and 12

BREAKFAST
Quinoa Berry Cereal

LUNCH
Rice, Tuna and Petits Pois Salad

DINNER
Chestnut and Mushroom Pilaf with steamed savoy cabbage
or leeks

Days 3, 8 and 13

BREAKFAST
Apricot Nut Shake and Tofu Scramble

LUNCH
Chestnut and Butter Bean Soup

DINNER
Poached Salmon and Sesame Steamed Vegetables
with Quinoa
Baked Apple with Spiced Blackberry Stuffing

Days 4, 9 and 14

BREAKFAST
Fruity Millet Flakes

LUNCH
Walnut and Three-Bean Salad

DINNER
Fast-and-easy Seasonal Stir-fry

Days 5 and 10

BREAKFAST
Sesame Rice Cereal

LUNCH
Pumpkin Seed Pesto with pasta★
Green Salad

DINNER
Cod Roasted with Lemon and Garlic, with steamed mixed
vegetables
Coconut Quinoa Pudding

★ Wheat-, gluten- and dairy-free – see **Note** with recipe

REINTRODUCING FOODS

Although much of this diet is consistent with an ongoing
healthy-eating regime, some foods have been excluded
because they cause allergic reactions in some people. These
foods may not necessarily be a problem for you, however. So,
once you've experienced the benefits of this diet over 14 (or
more) days, they can be reintroduced while monitoring any
changes in your symptoms using the method described in
Chapter 9. It is therefore best to introduce one food at a time

and to wait two days before adding the next food. If your symptoms get worse, continue to exclude this food.

These are the foods to reintroduce:

- Low-gluten grains: oats, barley, rye
- Citrus fruits: oranges, grapefruit, lemons, limes
- Nightshade family vegetables: tomatoes, potatoes, aubergine and peppers
- Cayenne pepper, paprika, chilli
- Peanuts, pistachio nuts
- Eggs

Introduce one food at a time. The first three are food families. So, if you are not sensitive to oats you probably won't react to the other grains. The same applies to citrus and nightshade-family vegetables.

Other foods on the 'exclude' list are best avoided on an ongoing basis or, at least, eaten infrequently. Neither wheat nor dairy products are advisable on a daily basis. The high gluten content of wheat is irritating to the digestive tract, even if you are not allergic to it. Dairy produce contains hormone residues not designed for human consumption and eating them regularly has not been shown to be beneficial for either arthritis or osteoporosis. Eating such foods no more than every fourth day reduces the risk of developing an allergic reaction, provided you are not already reacting to them.

GET A LOAD OFF YOUR JOINTS

There is little doubt that excess weight makes arthritis worse and joint damage more likely. Obesity has been associated with both osteoarthritis and rheumatoid arthritis, particularly in weight-bearing joints. A survey of 4,225 people with osteoarthritis found that obesity was definitely associated with osteoarthritis in the knees, particularly among women.[17] Physical examination of obese people found evidence of osteoarthritis in the knee even in people who had no evidence of knee pain. Frame size made little difference.

While the mechanical stress of excess weight on joints seems to be the major reason for the association between obesity and arthritis, other researchers have reported an association between obesity, inflammation and arthritis in non-weight-bearing joints, such as fingers.[18] Almost every overweight person has a degree of 'metabolic syndrome', also called syndrome X. This describes a collection of symptoms associated with losing blood sugar balance and increasing inflammation.

As well as paving the way for obesity, this syndrome is likely to disturb the balance of hormones controlling calcium levels in bone. It is more than likely that a high GL diet, low in natural anti-inflammatory nutrients, is the link between obesity and arthritis.

Whichever comes first, obesity or arthritis, once movement – and therefore exercise – is restricted it becomes harder to lose weight. Highly restrictive diets are unlikely to provide optimum amounts of all the nutrients that may lessen arthritis symptoms. However, by following the diet recommended in this book, which is designed to improve your metabolism and keep your blood sugar level even, weight can be lost without severe calorie restriction. The most effective weight-loss approach is a low glycemic-load (low-GL) diet (read my book, *The Low-GL Diet Bible*).

So, if you are overweight, follow the recommendations of the anti-arthritis diet strictly, reducing quantities as needed, and stick to a regular exercise regime that burns calories while not over-straining the joints (Chapter 25). Have the breakfast drink Get Up & Go (see page 257) five days out of seven, as this provides a high level of all nutrients and less than 300 calories – it's a great way to start the day.

SUMMARY

Aim to:

- **Maintain an even blood sugar level** by avoiding sugary, refined foods and stimulants, and eating pulses and wholegrains.
- **Eat smaller quantities of protein**, choosing higher quality sources, such as quinoa and soya.
- **Reduce your dairy consumption**, replacing cow's or goat's milk with soya milk.
- **Reduce your intake of saturated fat**, mainly found in meat, eggs and dairy produce.
- **Increase your intake of essential fats**, found in fish, nuts, seeds and their oils.
- **If you are overweight, follow a balanced, healthy diet** providing around 1,500 calories per day, and take regular exercise. The most effective weight-loss approach is a low glycemic load (low-GL) diet (read my *Low-GL Diet Bible*).
- **Eat plenty of fruit and vegetables**, as well as seeds, nuts, fish, herbs and spices (excluding chilli pepper, cayenne pepper and paprika).

CHAPTER 22

MY TOP ANTI-ARTHRITIS RECIPES

The following recipes will help you put the diet suggestions from Chapter 21 into practice. Once you've found out what you do and don't react to, you'll have a wider list of foods to choose from.

Almost all the recipes are sugar-free, using the natural sweetness present in food, or a natural plant sugar called xylitol that has all the taste of sugar but a third of the calories, and does not disrupt your blood sugar, giving it a very low GL (see page 73). Another added bonus is the fact that it protects your teeth from cavities (see Resources for suppliers).

Most of the lunches and main meals give quantities for two people. If there's only one of you, halve the portion sizes or make enough for two meals and pop one in the fridge.

Note I often suggest you season a dish with a little Solo sea salt, a special kind of salt that has half the sodium, and more magnesium and potassium than in regular salt (see Resources for more details).

Bon appétit!

BREAKFASTS

In addition to the suggestions below, it's worth checking to see whether your local health-food store stocks any suitable, ready-made cereals, such as puffed rice, puffed millet or gluten-free muesli. Just serve with soya milk, and some fresh fruit, if you wish.

A powerful breakfast: Get Up & Go

Nutritious Get Up & Go is a powdered breakfast drink, which is blended with skimmed milk or soya milk and banana or berries. Nutritionally speaking, it is the ultimate breakfast: each serving gives you more fibre than a bowl of porridge, more protein than an egg, more iron than a cooked breakfast and more vitamins and minerals than a whole packet of cornflakes. In fact, every serving of Get Up & Go gives you at least 100 per cent of every vitamin and mineral and a lot more of some key nutrients. For example, you get 1,000mg of vitamin C – the equivalent of more than 20 oranges.

Get Up & Go is made from the best-quality wholefoods, ground into a powder. The carbohydrate comes principally from apple powder, the protein comes from quinoa, soya and rice flour, the essential fats from ground sesame, sunflower and pumpkin seeds, the fibre from oat bran, rice bran and psyllium husks, and additional flavour from almond meal, cinnamon and natural vanilla.

It contains no sucrose, no additives, no animal products, no yeast, wheat or milk, and it tastes delicious. Each serving, with half a pint of skimmed milk or soya milk and some fruit, provides fewer than 300 calories and, when mixed up, only 10 GLs (see page 74). Get Up & Go is nutritionally superior to any other breakfast choice

continued

and is totally suitable for adults and children alike. It is fine to have this for breakfast every day, if you choose. It is widely available in health-food stores. (See Resources for stockists.)

Make Get Up & Go with berries such as strawberries, raspberries or blueberries, or a soft pear. If you use a banana, have a small, less ripe one or use half a larger banana.

GET UP & GO

This simple breakfast makes a wholesome start to the day.

SERVES 1

1 serving Get Up & Go powder
300ml (½ pint) skimmed milk or soya milk
1 small banana or a serving of other fruit (such as berries or peach)

Blend the milk, fruit and Get Up & Go powder, and serve.

QUINOA BERRY CEREAL

Quick, simple and satisfying, with all the goodness of the grain.

SERVES 2

75g (2¾oz) quinoa
soya milk (to taste)
a large handful of fresh blueberries
1 tsp flax seed oil

Put the quinoa in a pan with 400ml (14fl oz) water, and bring to the boil. Cover and simmer for 15–20 minutes, or until tender. Mix in the other ingredients and serve.

FRUITY MILLET FLAKES

This satisfying breakfast is a good source of fibre, as well as essential fats (the fats which are essential to our well-being, and can help 'oil' joints).

SERVES 1

1 tbsp millet flakes
apple juice (enough to cover millet flakes)
1 apple, grated
1 banana, chopped
1 tbsp mixed sunflower, pumpkin and sesame seeds
a pinch of ground mixed spice

Soak the millet flakes overnight in the apple juice. Combine with the other ingredients and serve.

SESAME RICE CEREAL

On a cold winter's day there's nothing more warming than porridge – this is porridge with a difference though. You just get some rice flakes from a health-food store and cook them as you would cook oats.

SERVES 1

300ml (½ pint) soya milk
25g (1oz) rice flakes
1 banana, sliced
1 tbsp ground sesame seeds

Put 300ml (½ pint) water and half the milk in a pan and sprinkle in the rice flakes. Bring to the boil and boil for 5 minutes, stirring all the time. Serve with the remaining soya milk, banana and ground seeds.

APRICOT NUT SHAKE

This dairy-free alternative to milkshake provides an instant and sustaining breakfast.

SERVES 1

50g (1¾oz) almonds
2 tbsp mixed sunflower and pumpkin seeds
6 fresh apricots, or use dried and soak overnight

Blend the nuts and seeds with 150ml (¼ pint) water until smooth. Add the apricots, blend again and serve.

TOFU SCRAMBLE

A great alternative to scrambled eggs.

SERVES 1

1 tsp olive oil
50g (1¾oz) shredded carrot
50g (1¾oz) chopped onion
100g (3½oz) firm tofu pieces
¼ tsp turmeric
chopped fresh parsley, to taste

Heat the oil in a frying pan and gently fry the carrot and onion until soft. Crumble the tofu and add to the pan, with the turmeric. Heat through, stirring until the tofu and vegetables are coated with seasoning. Just before serving, add the fresh parsley.

SALADS, SOUPS, DIPS AND LIGHT MEALS

Many of these recipes can be made and refrigerated, so, to save time you may want to make enough for two or three days. Most of these recipes would make great packed lunches for work, too.

Salads

Fresh vegetables tossed with a dressing and served with nuts, beans or tuna make excellent lunches and give your body a nutrient boost.

WALNUT AND THREE-BEAN SALAD

No foods are better than beans for satisfying your appetite and giving you stamina. It helps if they're served in a delicious, crunchy salad such as this one.

SERVES 2

400g (14oz) can mixed beans (such as haricots, chickpeas and
    flageolet), drained and rinsed
handful of walnuts, roughly chopped
½ apple, cubed
2 tsp fresh flat-leaf parsley or chives, chopped
1 tbsp olive oil
1 tbsp walnut oil or olive oil
juice of ½ lemon
1 celery stick, finely chopped
ground black pepper
Solo sea salt
mixed salad leaves, such as spinach, rocket and watercress, to serve

Combine all the ingredients and serve with the mixed salad leaves.

Rice, tuna and petits pois salad

This is unbelievably tasty – much more interesting than standard tuna mayo. Peas are delicious raw, and of course retain more vitamins this way.

SERVES 2

115g (4oz) brown basmati rice
115g (4oz) tuna in brine, drained and flaked
1 tsp sesame oil
2 tsp tamari or soy sauce
2 tsp lemon juice
1 tbsp fresh, uncooked petits pois
1 carrot, finely sliced lengthways into matchsticks
1 spring onion, finely sliced
ground black pepper

1 Cook the rice according to the pack instructions and allow it to cool.

2 Combine with all other ingredients, tossing thoroughly to mix all the flavours.

GREEN SALAD

This simple salad is a good accompaniment to any meal. It's subtly different because of the aniseed flavour from the fennel, and has plenty of crunch.

SERVES 4

1 Little Gem or other lettuce, torn into bite-sized pieces
¼ fennel bulb, finely sliced, or 2 tbsp fresh peas, uncooked (if you don't like fennel)
50g (1¾oz) broccoli tops, chopped
¼ cucumber, chopped
2 celery sticks, sliced
3 spring onions, sliced
1 tbsp French dressing (see below)

Combine all the ingredients in a bowl, toss with the French dressing and serve.

FRENCH DRESSING

This standard dressing can be jazzed up by adding fresh or dried herbs. You could also experiment with other oils such as cold-pressed sesame oil or flax oil, which contain essential fatty acids. Use as little dressing as possible on salads.

SERVES 4

2 tbsp Essential Balance Oil or Udo's Choice (from your local health food store), or olive oil
2 tbsp cider or balsamic vinegar
1 tsp French mustard
1 garlic clove, crushed

Put all the ingredients in a screw-top jar and shake vigorously. Add a little to salads. Any extra dressing can be stored in the fridge. It will keep for up to a month.

Soups

Warming and satisfying soups are always popular, and a home-made soup is so much tastier than shop bought – as well as being full of goodness.

CHESTNUT AND BUTTER BEAN SOUP

Chestnuts have the lowest fat content of all nuts and a pleasantly sweet flavour that goes well with the smooth texture of the butter beans.

SERVES 4

200g (7oz) cooked and peeled chestnuts (use vacuum-packed or canned)
1 onion, chopped
1 carrot, chopped
2 fresh thyme sprigs
1.2 litres (2 pints) vegetable bouillon or stock
400g (14oz) can butter beans, drained and rinsed
ground black pepper

1 Put all the ingredients except the butter beans in a large pan, cover and simmer very gently for 30 minutes. Add the beans, return to the boil and cook for 5 minutes.

2 Purée the soup until smooth and add black pepper.

BEANY VEGETABLE SOUP

This one-pot winter warmer is crammed full of fibre and is just the thing to take in a vacuum flask to work

SERVES 6

2 onions, chopped
3 celery sticks, finely chopped
3 leeks, sliced
450g (1lb) mixed root vegetables, such as carrot, swede and parsnip, peeled and chopped into bite-sized chunks
850ml (1½ pints) vegetable stock
2 400g (14oz) cans mixed pulses, or your choice of beans, such as kidney, chickpea, borlotti, butter or flageolet, drained and rinsed
fresh flat-leaf parsley, roughly chopped
Solo sea salt and ground black pepper

1 Put the onion, celery, leeks, root vegetables, stock and seasoning into a large pan and stir.

2 Cover and bring to the boil, then reduce the heat and simmer for 20 minutes.

3 Stir in the mixed pulses, then cover and simmer for 5–10 minutes, or until the vegetables are tender.

4 Add the parsley, then adjust the seasoning before serving.

THAI-STYLE VEGETABLE BROTH

This soup is packed with flavour and phytonutrients – and, even better, it tastes brilliant.

SERVES 4

4 thin slices of fresh root ginger, cut into thin matchsticks
2 garlic cloves, cut into thin matchsticks
600ml (1 pint) vegetable bouillon (Marigold Reduced Salt provides the best flavour for the soup base)
1 head pak choi, finely shredded
2 shiitake mushrooms, sliced
1 carrot, cut in half lengthways, then thinly sliced into half-moons
5 spring onions, sliced thinly at an angle
55g (2oz) firm tofu, cut into 1cm (½in) cubes
1 tbsp tamari or soy sauce

1 Put the ginger and garlic in a pan with the stock. Bring to the boil, cover and simmer for 3 minutes.

2 Bring the pan back to the boil and add the prepared vegetables and tofu. Season with the tamari, then reduce the heat and simmer for 3 minutes.

Dips

For a healthy snack or a simple lunch, make one of these quick and healthy dips to serve with sticks of celery, carrot and pepper as well as florets of raw broccoli or cauliflower.

HUMMUS

Chickpeas have a unique taste, which combines well with tahini, a paste of ground sesame seeds. You may prefer to buy ready-made hummus, which is widely available in supermarkets.

SERVES 2

400g (14oz) can chickpeas, drained and rinsed
2 garlic cloves, crushed
2 tbsp olive oil
juice of ½ lemon
2 tsp tahini
pinch of cayenne pepper
Solo sea salt

Put all the ingredients in a food processor or blender and whiz until smooth and creamy, adding a little water if necessary. Adjust the seasoning to taste.

FLAGEOLET BEAN DIP

This is an unusual, decorative and tasty alternative to hummus that is delicious on oatcakes or with crudités. It keeps in the fridge for two days.

SERVES 4

400g (14oz) can flageolet beans, rinsed and drained
5 spring onions
1 garlic clove, crushed
handful flat-leaf parsley, finely chopped
2 tbsp lemon juice
1 tbsp olive oil
1 tbsp water, if needed
Solo sea salt and ground black pepper

Put the beans, onions, garlic, parsley, lemon juice and oil into a blender, and blend until smooth. Add the water if necessary, then add the seasoning slowly, according to taste.

Light meals

When you want just a light bite in the evening, make these super-quick dishes that are full of flavour and nutrients.

HOT-SMOKED FISH WITH AVOCADO

The avocado provides healthy monounsaturated fat, while the fish gives plenty of omega-3 oils – just don't eat this more than once a week, to keep within your fat limit.

SERVES 2

2 fillets hot-smoked salmon or trout
5cm (2in) piece of cucumber, cut into bite-sized pieces
½ ripe medium-sized avocado
juice of 1 lemon
1–2 tsp chopped fresh dill or chives
1–2 tsp chopped fresh flat-leaf parsley
Solo sea salt and ground black pepper

1　Skin the fish and remove any bones, then flake into chunks. Put in a salad bowl with the cucumber.

2　Cut the avocado into bite-sized pieces. Add to the bowl together with the lemon juice and herbs. Season with Solo and pepper, and gently mix together.

COOK'S TIP
Leave the stone in the leftover half of avocado and drizzle with lemon juice to prevent discoloration, then cover and put in the fridge for future use.

PUMPKIN SEED PESTO

This keeps in the fridge for 2–3 days and can be stirred through soup or pasta (see note below), or added to bean salads. It makes a pleasant change from the basil-and-pine-nut variety.

SERVES 4

55g (2oz) raw pumpkin seeds
55g (2oz) flat-leaf parsley
55g (2oz) basil leaves
2 garlic cloves, crushed
1 tsp Solo sea salt
2 tsp lemon juice
55g (2oz) freshly grated Parmesan cheese
90ml (6 tbsp) pumpkin seed oil (roasted if you can find it) *or* the same
   quantity of pumpkin seed butter instead of the separate seeds and
   oil (available from Totally Nourish, see Resources)

1 Put the pumpkin seeds in a small blender or food processor with the herbs, garlic, salt, lemon juice and Parmesan. Whiz until the mixture is blended but retains some texture.

2 Add the pumpkin seed oil and mix until the pesto is an even consistency.

COOK'S TIP
There are many good wheat-, gluten- and dairy-free pastas available from most supermarkets or health-food stores – try Orgran Rice & Corn Pasta. It is best to get the spirals rather than the tubes, as tubes tend to fall apart when cooking. Cook the pasta according to the instructions (remembering not to overcook) and mix with the Pumpkin Seed Pesto. Top with basil, pumpkin seeds and black pepper and serve with a Green Salad.

MAIN MEALS

There are meals using chicken and fish here as well as vegetarian options, to give you a wide and healthy choice. Generally speaking, however, the recipes are designed for easy adaptation as far as protein is concerned, so you could substitute meat or fish for the vegetarian alternatives or substitute tofu, nuts or beans for meat or fish in the other recipes.

FAST-AND-EASY SEASONAL STIR-FRY

This is a healthier, lower-fat version of stir-frying. Versatility is the name of the game here, using a variety of sauces – from Chinese to Indian – and other ingredients: throw in cauliflower and sugar snap peas one night, carrots and mushrooms the next; use tempeh on Monday and chicken on Sunday – in short, anything goes. This is the perfect fallback recipe, using whatever's in the fridge and storecupboard for a truly tasty meal. The recipe ingredients are divided into vegetables, seasonings and protein-rich foods. Choose your selection and flavourings before you begin.

SERVES 2

Vegetables
spring onions, chopped
1 garlic clove, crushed
your choice from: carrots, broccoli, courgettes, cauliflower, sugar snap
    peas, runner beans, water chestnuts, mushrooms, beansprouts,
    bamboo shoots, enough to fill half each plate, cut into similar-sized
    thin pieces

Seasonings
Thai: 1 tsp green curry paste, a dash of coconut milk, a handful of
    chopped fresh coriander, added at the end of cooking
Chinese: 1 tsp tamari or soy sauce; 2.5cm (1in) fresh root ginger,
    finely chopped; 1 crushed garlic clove

Indian: 1 tsp ground coriander, 1 tsp ground cumin, ½ tsp ground
   turmeric
Japanese: 1cm (½in) fresh root ginger, finely chopped; tamari or soy
   sauce, teriyaki or yakitori sauce, to taste (try Kikkoman's, available in
   supermarkets)

Protein-rich foods
310g (11oz) tofu or tempeh, cubed
or 2 medium skinless chicken breasts, cut into strips
or 140g (5oz) filleted fish, cubed

1 Steam-fry the onion and garlic in your chosen seasoning.
   Add the protein-rich food and stir-fry until cooked (if using
   fish, stir-fry briefly until just cooked through and then
   remove from the pan).

2 Add your chosen vegetables, stir-fry briefly, then add 1 tbsp
   water and clamp on the lid. Steam until the vegetables are
   cooked but still crunchy. If using fish, return to the pan and
   heat through before serving.

Chicken and fish recipes

CHICKEN WITH ROASTED COURGETTES AND RED ONION

Roasting vegetables with chicken is a great idea, as the vegetables absorb the flavour of the chicken. This version uses a Mediterranean-inspired mix of courgette, sweet potatoes and red onion.

SERVES 2

2 courgettes, cut into chunks
2 red onions, cut into wedges
2 sweet potatoes, cut into 2.5cm (1in) dice
1½ tbsp olive oil
1–2 tbsp balsamic vinegar, according to taste
4 fresh thyme sprigs
2 garlic cloves, unpeeled
2 skinless chicken breasts
Solo sea salt and ground black pepper

1 Put the vegetables into a small roasting tin, pour over 1 tbsp of the oil and half the vinegar. Add a pinch of salt and the thyme. Toss together and put the chicken breasts on top, pressing them into the mixture so that they nestle between the vegetables.

2 Drizzle the remaining vinegar and oil over the chicken, and season.

3 Roast for 40–45 minutes at 180°C/350°F/Gas 4, shaking the vegetables around to recoat with oil and vinegar halfway through, and turning the chicken. Make sure it doesn't dry out on top.

TARRAGON AND LEMON ROAST CHICKEN BREAST

Fresh tarragon combined with garlic and lemon are favourite flavourings for roasted chicken. Cook the chicken breasts with the skin on to retain the moisture and flavourings, then remove the skin before serving.

SERVES 2

1 garlic clove, sliced
2 fresh tarragon sprigs
2 small chicken breasts (with skin)
2 tsp olive oil
½ lemon

1 Preheat the oven to 190°C/375°F/Gas 5. Insert the garlic slices and tarragon under the skin of the chicken.

2 Put the chicken breasts in a baking dish and drizzle with the olive oil and lemon juice.

3 Bake for 15–20 minutes, or until cooked through (this will depend on the thickness of the chicken). The flesh should be white with no pink juices. Before eating, remove the skin.

FISH IN AN ORIENTAL-STYLE BROTH

This dish is full of fresh, clean flavours and would be perfect for a special dinner.

SERVES 2

150ml (¼ pint) vegetable bouillon
2 tbsp mirin (Japanese rice wine, available from supermarkets)
2 tbsp tamari
1 small chunk of fresh root ginger, sliced
2 garlic cloves, crushed
2 lemon slices
2 fish fillets (haddock, plaice or cod)
55g (2oz) broccoli, broken into very small florets
55g (2oz) carrots, coarsely grated
55g (2oz) pak choi, finely shredded
4 spring onions, thinly sliced
½ tsp sesame oil

1 Put the stock, mirin, tamari, ginger, garlic and lemon in a wok and bring to the boil.

2 Measure the thickness of the fish fillets at their thickest points, then reduce the heat in the wok and slide the fish in. Poach for 10 minutes for every 2.5cm (1in) of thickness, or until the flesh turns opaque and flakes easily.

3 Lift the fish out of the broth and remove the skin, then divide the flesh between two soup bowls, cover and keep warm.

4 Bring the broth back to the boil and add the vegetables in the order listed, at 30-second intervals, cooking for a total of 2–3 minutes or until they are tender but very *al dente*. Remove the vegetables and add to the bowls.

5 Boil the broth for a further 30 seconds, then remove the ginger and lemon slices and stir in the oil. Ladle over the fish and vegetables, and serve immediately.

COD ROASTED WITH LEMON AND GARLIC

A delicious, no-fuss fish dish that is perfect for a light summer supper.

SERVES 2

½ tbsp olive oil
½ tbsp chopped fresh parsley
2 garlic cloves, crushed
2 cod fillets (or haddock or plaice)
1 lemon, thinly sliced
Solo sea salt and ground black pepper

1 Mix together the oil, parsley, garlic and seasoning, then rub over the fish. Set aside to marinate for 10 minutes. Preheat the oven to 180°C/350°F/Gas 4.

2 Put the fish on a baking tray and arrange the lemon slices on top. Bake for 8–10 minutes, or until just cooked through and the flesh flakes easily.

POACHED SALMON

Salmon responds well to extremely simple treatments, as in this recipe. Fast food with a difference!

SERVES 2

2 small salmon fillets
2 lemon wedges
Solo sea salt and ground black pepper

1 Put the salmon fillets in a shallow pan with just enough water to cover, and poach them gently for 15 minutes, or until just cooked through and the flesh flakes easily (timing will depend on the thickness of the fillets).

2 Season and serve garnished with lemon wedges.

Vegetarian recipes

CHESTNUT AND MUSHROOM PILAF

The flavours in this dish go together beautifully. To add a bit of colour, serve with steamed savoy cabbage or leeks.

SERVES 2

1 tbsp olive oil
55g (2oz) brown basmati rice
2 garlic cloves, crushed
2.5cm (1in) fresh root ginger, peeled and finely chopped
1 small onion, chopped
115g (4oz) shiitake or button mushrooms, sliced
150ml (¼ pint) stock made with Marigold vegetable bouillon
175g (6oz) cooked chestnuts (vacuum-packed or canned)
2 tsp tamari or soy sauce
55g (2oz) frozen peas

1 Gently heat the oil in a heavy frying pan and fry the rice for 3–4 minutes, or until it is pale brown. Add the garlic and ginger, stirring for 30 seconds, then add the onion and cook for a further 3 minutes. Add the mushrooms and cook for 3 minutes.

2 Stir in the stock, chestnuts and tamari or soy sauce, then cover and simmer for 35 minutes, or until the liquid is absorbed and the rice is just tender.

3 Stir in the frozen peas at the end and allow to cook gently and turn bright green before serving.

ROASTED VEGETABLES WITH MEDITERRANEAN QUINOA

Quinoa is amazingly versatile and very special, because it is packed full of protein. It's a great foil for these Mediterranean flavours.

SERVES 2

1 medium courgette, cubed
1 red onion, sliced into wedges
2 sweet potatoes, cut into wedges
1 handful of button mushrooms
4 tsp olive oil
Solo sea salt

For the quinoa
225g (8oz) quinoa
1 tsp vegetable bouillon or ½ stock cube
1 tbsp fresh basil leaves, finely chopped
4 stoned black olives (Kalamata preferably), roughly chopped
ground black pepper

1 Preheat the oven to 180°C/350°F/Gas 4. Put all vegetables on a baking tray, drizzle lightly with the olive oil and sprinkle with Solo. Toss to mix.

2 Bake for 40–50 minutes, or until all the vegetables are tender. Remove twice during cooking and shake the tray to turn and recoat the vegetables.

3 Meanwhile, rinse the quinoa very well under cold, running water. Put it in a pan with the bouillon powder or crumbled stock cube and 600ml (1 pint) water. Bring to the boil, cover and simmer for 13 minutes, or until the water has boiled away and the grains are light and fluffy.

4 Stir the basil and olives into the quinoa using a fork. Serve a mound of the quinoa topped with vegetables. Add freshly ground black pepper.

SESAME STEAMED VEGETABLES WITH QUINOA

Steaming vegetables brings out their individual delicate flavours, but the dressing in this recipe adds real pizzazz, turning them into a light, delicious feast.

SERVES 2

225g (8oz) quinoa
1 tsp vegetable bouillon or ½ stock cube
4 broccoli florets, chopped
2 handfuls of mangetouts
1 handful of baby corn
2 spring onions, chopped

For the dressing
2 tsp sesame oil
2 tsp tamari
1 tbsp sesame seeds, toasted in a dry pan until golden
a squeeze of lemon juice

1 Rinse the quinoa very well under cold, running water. Put into a pan with 600ml (1 pint) water and the bouillon or stock cube. Bring to the boil, then cover and simmer for 13 minutes, or until the water is absorbed. Fluff up the grains using a fork.

2 Put the broccoli in a vegetable steamer and steam for 4½ minutes. Add the mangetouts and baby corn, and cook for a further 2 minutes, or until the vegetables are just lightly cooked.

3 Mix all the dressing ingredients in a cup. Serve the vegetables on a mound of quinoa and pour the dressing over the top, then sprinkle with chopped spring onions.

DESSERTS

You can still eat healthily and enjoy a dessert. The recipes here are sweetened with a little xylitol to make them delicious without being oversweet and sugary, which is bad for your blood sugar level.

CINNAMON STEAMED PEARS WITH SUMMER BERRY PURÉE

Steaming is much easier than poaching these pears, which are lovely served with puréed summer berries.

SERVES 2

2 ripe pears
½ tsp cinnamon
1 tsp xylitol
2 heaped tbsp summer berries

1 Slice the bottom off each pear, so that they can stand unaided, then remove the core using either a melon–baller or a teaspoon.

2 Mix the cinnamon and xylitol together, then sprinkle into the hollow of each pear, where the core has been removed.

3 Lay the pears in a steamer pan and steam for 8–10 minutes, turning halfway through, until they are soft when pierced with a knife. (Do not stand them up or you will lose all of the sweet juices inside.)

4 While the pears are steaming, purée the summer berries in a blender or stew slightly in 1 tbsp water until they burst and release some juice.

5 Serve the pears still warm, standing upright, with a dollop of the fruit purée.

BAKED APPLE WITH SPICED BLACKBERRY STUFFING

A warming, fibre-rich pudding for autumn and winter. Blue-berries also taste lovely cooked with apples this way.

SERVES 2

1 heaped tbsp blackberries
¼ tsp cinnamon or ginger
2 tsp xylitol
2 cooking apples, cored to create a fairly large hole inside

1 Preheat the oven to 180°C/350°F/Gas 4. Put the berries in a bowl and mix with the cinnamon or ginger and xylitol.

2 Put the apples in an ovenproof dish or plate and stuff with the berry mixture.

3 Bake for 35–40 minutes, or until the apples are soft right the way through (test by inserting a skewer) but still standing (overcooking will cause the apples to collapse).

COCONUT QUINOA PUDDING

A high-protein, low-GL version of the comfort-food classic, rice pudding. This is not a glamorous-looking pudding but it does taste delicious.

SERVES 2

115g (4oz) quinoa, rinsed
150ml (¼ pint) soya milk
1 tbsp desiccated coconut
2 tsp xylitol

Put all the ingredients in a pan and bring to the boil, then reduce the heat, cover and simmer until the quinoa is cooked – the grains will look light and fluffy, and will be soft to the bite.

FRUIT JUICE JELLY

This all-natural jelly can be made from your favourite fruit juice, such as cranberry or freshly squeezed orange. Serve with fresh blueberries.

SERVES 6

2 level tsp agar-agar (vegetarian alternative to gelatine, available from
    health-food stores. Alternatively, use 4 level tsp powdered gelatine)
600ml (1 pint) fruit juice, at room temperature

If using agar–agar, soak it in 3 tbsp water in a pan, for 5 minutes if using agar–agar powder or for 10–15 minutes if using flakes. Dissolve over a medium heat, stirring constantly, then turn up the heat and boil for 2–3 minutes, stirring constantly.

Stir in the fruit juice and pour into a glass bowl or individual ramekins, and chill until set.

If using gelatine, put 3 tbsp water in a small pan, sprinkle over the gelatine and leave for 5 minutes, or until it becomes spongy, without stirring. Put the pan over a very low heat and wait for the water to become clear (without stirring or boiling).

Warm a quarter of the juice and add to the gelatine, stirring it in well, then add the remaining juice and pour into a bowl. Chill until set.

CHAPTER 23

SUPPLEMENTS FOR OSTEOARTHRITIS AND RHEUMATOID ARTHRITIS

Research shows that you can achieve far better results in alleviating arthritis with dietary changes plus supplements than with diet alone. Vitamins and minerals are much less toxic than drugs and are unlikely to have anything other than positive effects, provided you stay within the dosage guidelines given in this book. Many arthritis sufferers have reversed their condition and remained drug-free through a combination of diet, supplements, exercise and postural alignment.

The recommendations in this chapter should be read in conjunction with the chapters in Parts 2, 3 and 4 that are relevant to your particular condition. This will help you to choose the most appropriate supplements.

VITAMINS AND MINERALS

The best way to start is to take a good all-round multivitamin and mineral, as the nutrients work together. In the chart on pages 290–1 the 'basic level' is the amount to supplement on top of a good diet, assuming you will be following the dietary guidelines in this book. This basic level equates to, for example, a multivitamin and mineral supplement, taken twice a day, and three vitamin C (1,000mg) tablets. It may cost you daily as much as the price of a bar of chocolate, a bag of crisps, a cup of coffee, a fraction of a glass of wine or pint of beer, or two cigarettes. If you show this chart to a health-food-store assistant they should be able to find the easiest and cheapest way to meet these levels. On page 352 you'll find a list of reputable suppliers to choose from.

ESSENTIAL FATS

The next category of nutrients comprises the essential fats GLA and EPA. GLA can be derived from linoleic acid, and EPA from linolenic acid, both of which are high in seeds and their oil. So, if you are eating enough of these you may not 'need' to supplement extra GLA. However, few of us achieve enough EPA. Both, however, have been shown to help reduce inflammation and are well worth experimenting with. The best way to do this is to start with the maximum therapeutic level for one month; then, if that helps, reduce to the basic level and see if the improvement continues. GLA is found in evening primrose oil and borage oil – 500mg of evening primrose oil provides around 50mg of GLA. So the basic level is three 500mg capsules of evening primrose oil a day.

EPA and DHA are found together in fish oil. A capsule providing EPA is almost certain to provide DHA in the right proportion, so EPA and DHA come together: 3,000mg of fish oil will give you around 1,000mg of EPA. Again, start with the maximum therapeutic dose; then, if this helps, reduce to the basic level after a month. Alternatively, experiment with increasing oily fish in your diet.

Both GLA and EPA supplements are relatively expensive, but they are available on prescription from your GP. If you find they help, it is well worth discussing this with your doctor to see if you can get your supplies on prescription.

> **Your basic supplements:**
>
> **Basic level** A multivitamin and mineral supplement, taken twice a day, and three vitamin C (1,000mg) tablets
> **Also take** GLA (if needed): three 500mg capsules of evening primrose oil a day
> **And** 3,000mg of fish oil, to give you around 1,000mg of EPA (EPA and DHA come together)

THE THERAPEUTIC USE OF VITAMINS AND MINERALS

You may then wish to experiment with increasing your intake of some nutrients that have been shown to be particularly beneficial for certain types of arthritis. Start with vitamins B_3 and pantothenic acid (B_5) – both have proven effective for all kinds of arthritis and are relatively inexpensive. Try these for two months at the maximum therapeutic level. If this helps, reduce the dose and see if the benefit is maintained. If not, return to the higher dose. If there is no change in the two months, return to the basic dose.

Next, especially if you have rheumatoid arthritis or inflammatory problems, try increasing your levels of the antioxidant nutrients selenium, and vitamins C and E. Once again, increase your intake of these nutrients to the maximum therapeutic levels for one month. (If you get loose bowels on so much vitamin C, reduce your intake accordingly.) If this makes a difference, gradually lower the doses until you find the lowest level that maintains the benefit.

You can also experiment with increasing your intake of the other important minerals, including calcium, magnesium, zinc, iron, copper, manganese and chromium. The best starting point is to take a high-potency multi that's rich in minerals. But even so, it's hard to get enough calcium and magnesium. I often recommend an additional bone-friendly formula. But, before you do this, it is best to have a mineral test, such as a hair mineral analysis (available through a nutritional therapist, or see Resources, page 348 for test labs) in case you already have high levels of copper and iron, both of which can be harmful.

WHICH SUPPLEMENTS ARE BEST?

Not all supplements are equal, because some types of particular supplements are more easily used by the body than others. At the end of this section I list them in the order of availability to the body, but first I'll explain why this happens.

Most of the elements essential for health are supplied from food to the body as a compound, bound to a larger molecule within the food. This binding is known as chelation, from the Greek word *chela* (meaning a 'claw'). Some form of chelation is important, since unbound minerals can become bound to undesirable substances that remove minerals from the body (such as phytic acid in bran, tannic acid in tea and oxalic acid in spinach).

Best-absorbed minerals

Minerals can be absorbed more easily if they are attached to an amino acid or protein constituent. Such forms of minerals are called 'amino acid chelates' or 'organic' compounds (a chemical definition that has nothing to do with organic farming). Examples of amino acid chelates are methionates, aspartates and picolinates. Some so-called amino acid chelates are better than others. This depends on how well the mineral binds to the amino acid. If it is loosely bound it may separate during digestion. There is a patented process, called the Albion process, that guarantees a high-quality chelate, and this is used by some companies.

The best form of chelate really depends on how the body makes use of the mineral. For example, the iron in meat is in a chelated form that the body can use directly for making haemoglobin, a constituent of red blood cells. The superior results achieved with chromium picolinate are therefore probably due to it being in a more similar form to that which the body uses than other forms of the mineral.

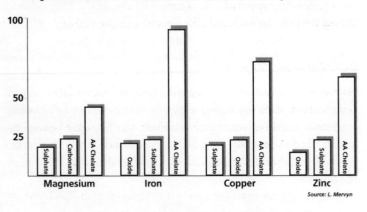

Chelates = amino acid chelates
Salts = oxides, sulphates or carbonates
% figures are differences in amounts absorbed, not amounts actually absorbed

Source: L. Mervyn

Figure 25 – Comparative absorption of different mineral compounds

The above shows that the chelated forms of magnesium, iron, copper and zinc are better absorbed than the salt forms; that is, oxides, sulphates or carbonates.

For some minerals, the extra cost of amino acid chelation outweighs the advantages. For example, calcium amino acid chelate is only twice as well absorbed as calcium carbonate, an inexpensive source of calcium. Iron amino acid chelate, on the other hand, is four times as well absorbed as ferrous oxide, making the price differential worth paying. Generally speaking, the following forms of minerals are most available to the body, listed in order of their bio-availability, so when choosing it's best to go for the first ones in each list if possible:

Calcium and magnesium – amino acid chelate, gluconate, citrate, carbonate

Iron – amino acid chelate, gluconate

Zinc – picolinate, amino acid chelate (for example, iron bisglycinate), citrate, gluconate

Chromium – picolinate, polynicotinate, amino acid chelate, gluconate

Selenium – amino acid chelate (for example, cysteine or methionine compound), gluconate

Manganese – amino acid chelate, citrate, gluconate

Best-absorbed vitamins

As far as vitamins are concerned, there is less variation from type to type. Vitamin C, for example, can be taken as ascorbic acid or calcium, or magnesium ascorbate, the latter being less acidic. Large amounts of calcium ascorbate should not be taken at mealtimes, since this may reduce the level of acid in the stomach and cause digestive problems.

The natural form of vitamin E, called d-alpha tocopherol (or tocopheryl), is preferable to its synthetic form, dl-alpha tocopherol, as it is 30 per cent more potent.

Vitamin B_3 is best in the 'non-blushing' niacinamide form, and B_5 as calcium pantothenate. Vitamin B_6 (pyridoxine) has to be converted into the active form known as pyridoxal-5-phosphate (P-5-P) before it can be used by the body. The enzyme that does this is zinc-dependent. So, for best utilisation of vitamin B_6, either take pyridoxal-5-phosphate itself, or take B_6 with zinc. Supplements are available that contain, for example, 100mg of B_6 and 10mg of zinc.

OPTIONAL EXTRAS

Finally, there are optional extras you may like to try, listed in the chart below, with suggested doses. The ones I would recommend first are curcumin and boswellia (if inflammation is involved) and glucosamine (for rebuilding healthy joints). Start with the maximum therapeutic level for one month. If any of these have a positive effect, reduce to the basic level and see if the improvement continues.

Many natural anti-inflammatory remedies available today are a combination of these nutrients. Each of us is individual and you will probably find that some of the above work better for you than others, so it is generally a case of experimenting. In terms of supplements you are best using formulas that combine some of these ingredients, in which case the dose needed of each individual ingredient may be less. Since their effect is probably synergistic, this may prove more effective than just taking one ingredient alone. They can also be found in creams that can be applied locally, reducing pain and swelling in specific joints (see page 55 and the Supplement, Remedy and Supplier Directory, under Resources, page 348, which lists supplements that contain a combination of many of these nutrients).

Optimum Anti-arthritis Supplement Intake

Nutrient	Basic Level	Maximum Therapeutic Level
Vitamins:		
A – beta-carotene/retinol	2,500mcg	
C – ascorbic acid	**2,000mg**	**10,000mg**
E – d-alpha tocopherol	**250mg**	**400mg**
D – cholecalciferol (D$_3$)	15mcg	45mcg
K – phylloquinone	50mcg	300mcg
B$_1$ – thiamine	25mg	
B$_2$ – riboflavin	25mg	
B$_3$ – niacinamide	**50mg**	**1,000mg**
B$_5$ – pantothenic acid	**50mg**	**1,000mg**
B$_6$ – pyridoxine	50mg	
B$_{12}$ – cyanocobalamine/ methylcobalamine	10mcg*	
Folic acid	100mcg	
Biotin	50mcg	
Minerals:		
Boron	1mg	3mg
Calcium	**300mg**	**600mg**

continued

Nutrient	Basic Level	Maximum Therapeutic Level	
Magnesium	**300mg**	**600mg**	
Iron	10mg		
Zinc	**10mg**	**35mg**	
Copper	1mg	3mg	
Manganese	2.5mg	25mg	
Selenium	**100mcg**	**200mcg**	
Chromium	50mcg	200mcg	
Essential fats:			
GLA	150mg	300mg	
EPA	**1,000mg**	**2,000mg**	
DHA	200mg	600mg	
Amino acids and other nutrients:			
IsoOxygene (hop extract)	500mg	1,500mg	anti-inflammatory
Hydroxytyrosol (Olivenol)	100mg	400mg	anti-inflammatory
Glucosamine	**1,000mg**	**2,000mg**	**cartilage building**
Mussel extract	250mg	1,000mg	cartilage building
Chondroitin	1,000mg	2,000mg	cartilage building
Glutamine	1,000mg	5,000mg	intestinal permeability
Curcumin	**500mg**	**1,500mg**	**anti-inflammatory**
Boswellia	**400mg**	**1,200mg**	**anti-inflammatory**
Ashwagandha	**300mg**	**600mg**	**anti-inflammatory**
MSM	**1,000mg**	**3,000mg**	**anti-inflammatory**
Quercetin	300mg	600mg	anti-inflammatory
Ginger extract	500mg	2,000mg	anti-inflammatory
Bromelain	200mg	400mg	anti-inflammatory
DLPA	750mg	2,250mg	pain control
S-adenosyl-methionine (SAMe)	00mg	1,200mg	pain control

The most important nutrients are shown in **bold**.
*1,000mcg if your homocysteine is high – methylcobalamine is the best-absorbed form.
Note The B vitamins are listed individually, so these are the amounts you should look for in a complex or a multi. It is advisable to take them in combination not isolation (unless advised by a nutritional therapist or nutritionally oriented doctor).

SAFETY FIRST

All the levels of nutrients recommended in this book fall well below the lowest levels at which adverse or toxic reactions have been reported. Please do not exceed the maximum therapeutic levels unless under the guidance of a qualified nutritional therapist (see Resources, page 344, to find one in your area) or a doctor. They can often speed up the process of helping you find the most effective supplement regime. If, in any event, you experience any adverse reactions that persist for more than three days, stop taking whatever you suspect is causing them and consult a qualified nutritionist or your doctor.

KNOWING WHAT WORKS

To find out what works for you, it is best to approach it scientifically. In other words, change one thing at a time, give it long enough to have an effect, and monitor any changes. For most nutrients, one month is the shortest and two months the longest period you need to find out if something is likely to help you.

Once you've been on your basic vitamin and mineral programme, add one extra item at a time so that you know what it is that makes a difference. If a nutrient does help, add it to your basic programme and then experiment with something else. Don't keep taking 'maximum therapeutic levels' of something that shows no clear result.

Chapter 26 explains how to monitor your improvement and keep a good record of your experiments with these different nutrients. These records will help any practitioner you may consult at a later date, so don't throw them away.

WHEN TO TAKE SUPPLEMENTS

Vitamins, minerals, essential fats and amino acids all work together in the body, so it is best to take additional supplements of nutrients with food, with the exception of bromelain (which is best taken between meals). The enzymes produced in the digestive tract also help to break down the protein coating on some supplements when you take them with your meals. However, if taking supplements twice or three times a day might mean that you forget the second or third lot, it is probably best to take them all at once. Here are the 'ten commandments' of supplement taking:

1 Take vitamins and minerals during a meal or within 15 minutes of eating.
2 Take most of your supplements with your first meal of the day.
3 Don't take B vitamins late at night if you have difficulty sleeping.
4 Take multiminerals or calcium/magnesium tablets in the evening – these help you sleep.
5 If you are taking two or more B complex or vitamin C tablets, take one at each meal.
6 Don't take individual B vitamins unless you are taking a B complex, or a combination of B vitamins within a multi-vitamin, and also make sure you don't exceed the maximum therapeutic dose of any one B vitamin in your overall daily dose. This is because B vitamins work synergistically.
7 Don't take extra individual minerals unless you are also taking a multivitamin.
8 If you are anaemic (iron-deficient) take extra iron with vitamin C.
9 If you know you are copper-deficient, take copper with only ten times as much zinc (for example 0.5mg copper to 5mg zinc).
10 Take your supplements every day. Irregular supplementation does not work.

Most of the natural remedies, from curcumin to quercetin, work best taken three times a day. So, divide your daily dose and take one-third with each main meal.

CHAPTER 24

MANAGEMENT AND PREVENTION OF BACK PAIN

Up to 80 per cent of us will suffer with the misery of back pain at some point in our life. As well as causing pain and discomfort, back pain costs billions in National Health Service treatment in the UK, and lost business revenues each year. Back pain can also be a symptom of arthritis. Bad posture and an inactive lifestyle, for example, can put pressure on the vertebrae causing back pain. Similarly, foot problems or incorrect footwear can affect your posture, creating arthritic problems in the future. Understanding why back pain occurs – and how you can keep your back in good shape – can help to reduce your risk of suffering.

THE MAIN CAUSES OF BACK PAIN

There can be a number of reasons why back pain occurs and most of them are connected to lifestyle: inactivity, being unfit, incorrect posture and being overweight, for example.

Inactivity

According to Clive Lathey, a leading osteopath with over 25 years of experience, the leading cause of back pain is sedentary living. He has helped tens of thousands of patients find relief from back pain and links the dramatic increase in recent times to the long periods of time many of us spend sitting at desks and computers, driving vehicles, flying and generally being less active.

The human spine is a complex piece of engineering which is designed to be active. Prolonged sitting places our spinal discs under strain. The discs are like shock absorbers between our vertebrae and have a 'jelly-like' substance inside them. A slumped sitting posture, which reverses the natural curve of the lower back, can increase disc pressure by as much as 190 per cent. This gradually weakens the tough spinal ligaments and outer layer of the disc, and subsequently can lead to the development of disc bulging (also known as a 'slipped disc').

Reduced fitness levels

If you live an inactive lifestyle with a sedentary job, it goes without saying that your overall body function will suffer. For example, in a typical day an average person may spend 30 minutes walking to and from public transport to their workplace and home again (and even less if they drive to work). The rest of the day, for the majority of people, will be spent inactive sitting at a desk. This may easily mean seven-to-ten hours of very little movement.

Mechanically, you will develop generally less flexible muscles and poor muscle tone, alongside increased joint stiffness. The spinal muscles will not only shorten and tighten, but also waste, which is known as muscle atrophy. The result of this is less ability to control and maintain body position, co-ordinate movements and maintain the natural 'S' shape of the spine. All these factors increase the likelihood of injury to your spine.

Bad posture

The way you hold your body is probably the most important factor in determining the health of your back. Poor posture will gradually weaken your back and result in pain.

Good posture is achieved by maintaining the S shape of the spine, both in a sitting or standing position (see the exercises to help you achieve this, pages 298–300). When the spine is in the S-shaped position, the centre of gravity is located in the mid-line or neutral location. In other words, the weight of your body is distributed equally along the length of the spine. In this position, the muscles in the front and back of the body are well toned, but relaxed.

A poor, slumped or C-shaped posture (particularly in sitting), will weaken the spinal discs, stretch ligaments and joints, tighten muscles and eventually cause pain.

Excess body weight

People who are overweight or obese are more likely to suffer with joint pain. Excess body weight not only leads to an increase in loading of many of the body's joints – which can contribute to the early wear and tear in arthritis – but also puts a tremendous strain on the back and neck.

The spine – with all its discs, muscles and ligaments – and the pelvis have to support the rest of the body. So, if there is extra weight, which generally pulls the body forward, all the components of the spine have to work very hard to maintain an upright posture. This means there is a much greater risk of a slipped disc, muscle tears and ligament sprains.

Overweight people often complain of lower back, knee, hip, ankle and foot pain. The body requires optimal health in order for damaged tissue to repair quickly and permanently. However if, as is often the case with obesity, the body is not in a healthy state, these tissues can become chronically damaged, resulting in long-term pain and reduced quality of life.

Congenital conditions

A number of people who complain of hip, back and neck pain have a spinal scoliosis (curvature of the spine), which may be the root cause, or at least a contributory cause, of the pain. The scoliosis may be due to other factors such as leg length difference or pelvic torsion, and so the spine tries to accommodate these asymmetries by twisting and rotating. In some people, the scoliosis may have occurred at birth, or later in life through a traumatic incident or long-term postural problems.

The consequences of a scoliotic spine will be uneven stresses and strains being placed upon the vertebral joints, discs, ligaments and muscles, resulting in damage and discomfort of varying degrees.

An osteopath can assess the type and degree of scoliosis, together with the possible causes and contributory factors. They can then perform manual treatment with the intention of minimising the scoliosis and/or assisting the body to adapt to the strains and thus reduce the pain. Postural advice and exercise regimes can also help in a rehabilitative and preventative manner.

WHAT SHOULD YOU DO IF YOU HAVE BACK PAIN?

Firstly, if you develop acute back pain, it is always advisable to consult a medical expert such as an osteopath, physiotherapist or your GP. There are simple clinical tests that can be done to clearly identify whether the back pain you are suffering from is of a serious nature or a simple mechanical problem.

Certain conditions such as rheumatoid arthritis, spondylolisthesis (vertebral slippage), fractures, slipped discs or compression in the nerves or spinal column need to be diagnosed and treated early to avoid any serious long-term injury to your spine, spinal cord and peripheral nerves. So, if in doubt, seek advice first and foremost.

The treatment of back pain usually follows a three-stage process. Firstly, reducing inflammation and pain. This is where nutrition can play a big role, so follow the recommendations given in Part 2. Secondly, restoring mobility. This is where an osteopath can often correct the initial problem through manipulation of soft tissues and mobilisation. Finally, the focus shifts to restoring stability and strength. This is a more long-term approach, which builds in a preventative aspect to the treatment. It may include an exercise regime, Pilates/core stability recommendations, postural changes, workstation advice and any other lifestyle changes that can positively benefit you.

For more complicated conditions, osteopaths often work alongside GPs or hospital consultants to ensure that you receive optimal care from both osteopathic and orthodox disciplines. For example, scans, blood tests and other investigations may be carried out by a GP or hospital and can aid diagnosis and help in determining the best treatment plan. This may include osteopathy, physiotherapy and certain medications. Again, a long-term programme is the best way to encourage optimal health.

Working at an ergonomically designed workstation with a chair that provides lower back support can help maintain a healthier spine, as can postural awareness and doing some regular and appropriate exercise.

EXERCISES THAT CAN BE HELPFUL FOR BACK PAIN

An episode of pain and immobility weakens the 'spinal core muscles', hence it is crucial that treatment is followed by a rehabilitation exercise programme. There are some very simple exercises to help you develop muscles that build core strength and improve your overall posture generally.

Standing exercise

1 Starting at your feet, try to stand with the weight going through both the heels and balls of your feet. Next, gently

draw in your tummy button towards your spine. At the same time gently lift your chest up and outwards, while moving your shoulders down and back.

2 Gently elongate your neck and bring your chin in towards your spine. Imagine a cord is gently lifting your head upwards from the crown.

Sitting exercise

1 Try to sit well back into the chair with your lower back supported and your weight evenly distributed on both buttocks and thighs. Your knees should be lower than your thighs. Do not sit with your legs crossed (if you have to, only do so for short periods of time). Keep your feet planted on the ground, hip-width apart if possible.

2 The shoulders should be down, back and relaxed and the head held straight, with the chin gently pulled in towards the spine (not poked forward). Do not sit for more than 30 minutes – aim to get up and walk around. Never cradle the telephone between your ear and shoulder, as this puts a lot of strain on your back and neck.

Other back exercises

These simple daily exercises can help to strengthen your back, stretch out tight muscles and aid improved posture. Do not continue with any exercises if you feel any pain.

Flexion stretch Lie on your back with your head on the floor, pull one knee to your chest and hold for a few seconds. Repeat with other leg. Repeat.

Back extension Lie face down with your hands on the floor, under your shoulders. Straighten your arms to push the top half of your body upwards. Hold for a few seconds and feel the stretch in your lower back. Slowly return to the floor. Repeat.

Flexion stretch 2 Start on all fours, then bend your knees and lower buttocks to your heels, and hold for a few seconds. Repeat.

Back stabilisation Start on all fours and, with a flat back and straight neck, stretch out your left arm and right leg simultaneously, and hold for a few seconds. Repeat with your right arm and left leg extended. Repeat.

General exercise

Research shows that 'cross training' – that is, mixing specific gym exercises (using gym equipment or floor exercises) with your chosen sport – helps reduce injuries. For example, playing tennis on one day and practising Pilates another, or running alternating with swimming, football with visits to the gym. This is because doing regular 'core' exercises (building up the abdominal, buttock and spinal muscles) in conjunction with other sports improves balance, posture and performance.

Pilates is particularly good for backs, as it is very muscle specific and involves flexibility and posture control. Yoga, t'ai chi, gyrotonics, walking/hiking and swimming can also be beneficial.

Footwear

Your feet support your body, so looking after them and choosing supportive footwear can help to promote a healthy back too. When exercising, wearing appropriate footwear is important; for example, wearing supportive training shoes that can absorb the shock of impact when walking, jogging or running.

For women, high heels worn long term can create a shortening of the calf and posterior thigh muscles, which can lead to muscle tension and damage. The body's centre of gravity is also thrown forward so that more pressure is exerted on the front of the feet, front of the knees and low back, as it attempts to keep you upright. These resultant forces over time can contribute to early arthritic changes to feet, knees, hips and the back. It is therefore only advisable to wear high heels for short periods at a time and as infrequently as possible. Wear trainers or a good supportive shoe to and from work and, if necessary, change into work shoes – but limit your use of high heels if you are standing all day.

Remember that shortened muscles are prone to injury while performing other activities such as walking, running, or gym sessions – but the damage has already been done by the high heels.

If you suffer with other foot problems such as overpronation (collapsed arch) or supination (very high arch), these can contribute to foot, ankle, knee, hip and back pain. An orthotic device can help restore balance and improve posture. There are also manipulative techniques that can improve the function of the feet, and these can be carried out by an osteopath.

For further information about Clive Lathey's osteopathic practice, or if you would like to find an osteopath in your area, see Resources, page 345.

CHAPTER 25

YOUR HYDROTHERAPY AND EXERCISE PROGRAMME

Exercise and hydrotherapy are a vital part of any anti-arthritis programme. The key is setting yourself a realistic routine and sticking to it. For the first few weeks you may need to exercise your will as well as your body, but, once established, exercising becomes as much of a habit as not exercising.

In this chapter I'll explain a little more about the benefits of exercise and where you can find some that will be best for your particular needs. Later in the chapter you will find a weekly exercise programme for you to follow.

STRENGTH, SUPPLENESS AND STAMINA

There are three important aspects to exercise: strength, suppleness and stamina. We need strength to function and to give support to the body, and strengthening exercises also help to increase bone density. Suppleness of muscles and joints declines with age, unless you exercise. Naturally, the joints you exercise the least become less supple. Your muscles may be compensating for bad posture, paving the way for problem areas later in life. Exercise also develops stamina by making demands on the heart and cardiovascular system to supply oxygen and nutrients to the working muscles. Increased stamina means decreased risk of cardiovascular disease.

Different kinds of exercise involve different amounts of these three key factors. Yoga is excellent for suppleness. Brisk walking is good for stamina. Gardening and physical hobbies are often good for strength. And swimming is good for all three.

THE BENEFITS OF EXERCISE

If you still think that eating the right diet is enough, consider this study by Bill Solomon from the University of Arizona, who decided to find out which was more important for health – diet or exercise.[19] He got some obliging pigs to run around a track but fed them the average, vitamin-deficient diet. Another group had the pig-equivalent of health-food but no exercise. A third group of pigs both exercised and ate a healthy diet. The third group did best overall, proving – predictably enough – that both exercise and diet are important.

Regular exercise also has many specific benefits in relation to arthritis. It supplies nutrients to the joints, lubricates and nourishes them, strengthens bones, increases mobility, decreases pain and stiffness, relaxes muscles, and reduces joint strain by keeping your weight down. On top of all that, it keeps your heart, arteries and lungs healthy, and improves energy and sleep.

ANTI-ARTHRITIS EXERCISES

Exercise is an important part of any anti-arthritis programme. Through exercise, joints are nourished and kept mobile. Because cartilage does not have a blood supply it relies on movement of the joint to stimulate a supply of nutrients. Resistance exercise increases bone density, helping to prevent osteoporosis, as explained in Chapter 17. Weightlessness studies at NASA have found that, in the absence of gravity, bones start to degenerate. Just walking around exercises muscles.

Bone density increases with weight-bearing exercise – unless you are a bear: research has shown that the bones of hibernating bears actually become more dense. It appears that, unlike us, a sleeping bear recycles its own calcium, rather than losing it.

In a clinical trial, the effects of exercise on bone mineral content were compared with the effects of supplementing 750mg of calcium and 400iu of vitamin D over a three-year period. The elderly women on this trial did 30 minutes of mild physical exercises while sitting in a chair, three times a week. At the end of the trial their bone mineral content had increased by 2.29 per cent, while those on supplements alone had increased by 1.58 per cent. Those doing no exercise and taking no supplements had a decrease in bone mineral content of 3.29 per cent. This study illustrates just how important exercise is for bone strength.[20]

Moderate exercise also boosts the immune system. T'ai chi was shown to increase T-cell count (needed for immunity) by 40 per cent. However, over-training or vigorous exercise can actually depress immune function.[21]

Exercise for arthritis – the golden rules

It is very important not to over-exercise or wrongly exercise affected joints – take great care not to overstress these. It is not necessary to feel pain for exercise to do you good, nor is it advisable. Of course, there is sometimes a degree of pain, especially after exercising muscles that have long been inactive. A good guideline is that if you experience pain induced by exercise for more than two hours afterwards, you are working too hard. Do a little less next time.

You can also protect yourself from unnecessary strain from certain exercises. For example, if you like walking

continued

or jogging, get a really supportive pair of shoes and walk on grass rather than on the road. Rebounders (mini-trampolines) are a great way of reducing strain on the knees and hips. They are available from the Wholistic Research Company (see Resources, page 346). Exercise practised in water is the best of all. Many anti-arthritis exercises can be done either in the bath or in a swimming pool.

Osteoarthritis benefits most from regular exercise that strengthens affected joints and increases their flexibility. Improved strength supports the joint, while flexibility discourages the formation of spurs. Both nourish the joint by increasing circulation of fluid.

Rheumatoid arthritis requires care. Rheumatic joints benefit most from periods of rest and periods of exercise. Over-exercising can cause flare-ups, which are to be avoided. If joints are actively inflamed and are hot and painful, they should not be vigorously exercised, although they can be passively taken through their range of movement at different times during the day. Yoga exercises are particularly good here. However, when your joints aren't inflamed it's important to exercise them and develop some strength.

A word of caution If a joint is aching or inflamed, either perform very light, loosening exercises that take the joint through its range of motion, or rest the joint completely. Make sure you do not overstress any aching joint. Know your body's limitations and do not cause yourself unnecessary pain. This will slow down your healing, not speed it up. Use cold compresses to calm down a hot, inflamed joint.

FINDING THE RIGHT EXERCISES

A physical-health professional can recommend specific exercises for you to carry out, but exercises for each body area are also given in a number of excellent books. The two I particularly recommend are *Exercise Beats Arthritis* by Valerie Sayce, and *Office Yoga* by Julie Friedberger (see Recommended Reading). There is also a booklet with exercises available from Arthritis Care. Hatha yoga and Psychocalisthenics also contain a number of exercises that can be adapted to suit your needs. When you have decided on the exercises that are best for you, follow an exercise programme – I'll show you how.

YOUR EXERCISE AND HYDROTHERAPY PROGRAMME

Think of exercise as one of the natural remedies you are employing to cure your arthritis. No doubt you will follow a diet and take supplements virtually every day. The same thing applies to exercise. You need to establish a routine and stick to it.

Aim for at least 15 minutes' exercise each day. This may increase to 30 minutes. Two days a week it may be swimming, two days a week it may be a walk, leaving three days a week to do a routine at home.

Pick a time in the day, preferably when you feel good, not exhausted. Make sure you will not be disturbed, so that you can have 15–30 minutes of peace, simply exercising – this in itself is calming. Joints and muscles benefit most from exercise once they have been stretched and 'warmed up'. It's good to warm up by doing some simple exercises that take joints through their range of movement. You may wish to start by focusing specifically on one problem area. This is quite useful in that you can soon get a sense of what effect regular exercise has on a set of joints. Ultimately it is better, however, to exercise the whole body. End your exercise session with some simple stretches, much like the warm-up. This helps to maintain the flexibility you have created while exercising.

After exercising is a great time to take a bath or apply one of the hydrotherapy techniques discussed in Chapter 13.

The following programme provides a good basis, which you should adapt to suit your own lifestyle. Monitor your progress, as explained in Chapter 26.

DAYS 1 AND 4: STRETCH INTO STRENGTH AND SUPPLENESS

These are your suppleness-and-strength exercise days. Make sure, over the two days, that you exercise all the areas listed and their related joints. Exercise arthritic or aching joints in both sessions. Initially, aim for 15 minutes. Then build this up to 30–60 minutes. These exercises are generally best done in the morning or evening.

Warm up

Start each session with warm-up exercises to relax, lengthen and bring circulation to the muscles you are about to work. Then, very gently stretch each part of your body, not pulling any muscle or joint further than it will comfortably go. Hold each stretch for 20 seconds and release.

Another great way to do this is to start with a warm shower, then turn the tap to cold. Shower each area of your body that is affected, rubbing the area with your hands and mentally becoming conscious of it, saying inwardly 'I bring conscious-ness to my knees/hands', and so on. The cold water brings energy to the joint, which responds with a warm glow. Follow this with your warm-up exercises, then your stretches.

Stretching exercises

A great way to develop suppleness and strength in all these areas is to join a yoga class and get some specific instruction from your yoga teacher. Another exercise system that can be very helpful is called Psychocalisthenics (see Resources, page 345). It takes a day to learn and, once learnt, you can do the simple 20-minute routine at home. However, go easy on the exercises that are hard for you. Again, ask an instructor for some personal guidance so that you can adapt the exercise regime to fit your own requirements, depending on any disability you may have. Yoga is preferable for the severely disabled, but it is best to do this under the guidance of a specialist yoga instructor.

Cool down

To cool down, again gently stretch out each set of muscles. Then lie on the floor on your back, imagining each part of your body – from your toes to your head – relaxing, one after the other. You can mentally say to yourself, 'I relax my toes, I am relaxing my toes, my toes are completely relaxed' for each part.

Programme for Days 1 and 4

1 Shower (hot and cold) before and/or after your exercise session
2 Warm up
3 Neck exercises
4 Arm exercises
5 Hand exercises
6 Back exercises
7 Knee exercises
8 Feet exercises
9 Cool down

DAYS 2 AND 6: BUILDING UP STAMINA

These days are for building stamina through aerobic exercise, which, by definition, needs to be hard work and make your heart beat faster. Good examples are swimming, walking, cycling, stair-climbing or attending an exercise or dance class. Whatever you choose, make sure the exercise is low impact and doesn't over-strain your joints. Invest in a good pair of shoes and don't over-stretch yourself.

Aim for 15 minutes to start with, then build up to 30–60 minutes depending on the kind of exercise. Swimming for 15 minutes, for example, is equivalent to more than half an hour of brisk walking. A good routine is to swim once a week and walk once a week. As with Days 1 and 4, start each session with warm-up exercises and end each session with cool-down exercises.

After each aerobic exercise session have a soothing warm bath, adding 100g (3½oz) of sodium bicarbonate (which you can buy in any chemist). Acid by-products are produced when muscles work hard. Sodium bicarbonate has an alkalising effect and reduces muscle stiffness.

Programme for Days 2 and 6

1 Aerobic exercise
2 Alkalising bath

DAYS 3 AND 7: MASSAGE AND RELAXATION

If you can, it is well worth having a therapeutic massage once a week or once a fortnight. This can help to improve healing and circulation, and to relax traumatised muscles. It's good to have a massage therapist recommended to you. Otherwise, contact a reputable health centre near you.

Alternatively, you can learn how to give yourself a massage. Self-massage is the highest form of healing, since it is you directing your will to heal yourself. Some areas of the body, however, are rather hard to reach. It is a good idea to have an alkalising bath after such a massage as well.

Programme for Days 3 and 7

Massage and relaxation

DAY 5: ENJOYMENT

Leave one day a week completely free of any routine. Relax and enjoy yourself. Since it is a good idea to exercise three days out of seven, go for a swim or a walk or some other activity that exercises but doesn't over-strain the body.

Programme for Day 5

Relax and enjoy yourself

SETTING GOALS AND STICKING TO THEM

Once you've worked out what you have to do to maintain suppleness, strength and stamina, you need to stick to it! It's essential to plan your programme, write it down and monitor your progress. Draw up a routine, Monday to Sunday, that you can follow. Don't be over-ambitious. Ask yourself honestly if the goals you have set are realistic and achievable. It is much better to succeed at a low-level programme than to fail and ditch exercise altogether. When you've worked out a viable and effective routine, display it somewhere obvious and consult it every day.

If you miss your exercise sessions for a few days when other events take over, remember to get back to the programme. I remind myself at the beginning of each week to follow my routine. Whatever I did yesterday or last week becomes irrelevant. What *is* relevant is doing my routine scheduled for today. The guidelines in Chapter 26 will help you monitor your progress.

CHAPTER 26

MONITORING YOUR PROGRESS

Monitoring your progress in a systematic way has two advantages. The first is that you are more likely to find out which factors make a difference to your arthritis. Too often people embark on a new regime that contains some pieces of advice that help them whereas other pieces of information don't. For example, a diet that excludes all common allergens may help, but, unless you investigate how you feel with or without specific foods, you may end up eating an unnecessarily restrictive diet. The second advantage of monitoring is that it helps you stick to your chosen regime.

MONITORING CHANGE

The first step in monitoring your condition is to pick specific symptoms that may change, such as pain, joint flexibility, morning stiffness, swelling or general lack of energy. Pick three or four symptoms that you can genuinely rate as 'better' or 'worse' from week to week. For example, if you have no pain, give 'pain' a Health Rating of 100 per cent. If you have unbearable pain, give it a Health Rating of 0 per cent. What is the worst you've ever been? Where are you now?

Pick a time, perhaps on Sunday, when you can look back over the week and assess whether your pain has been worse or better (you may be able to do this by keeping a record of how often you use painkilling drugs, if you do). If you started at 30 per cent and have improved a little, rate your pain level at 40 per cent.

The following Sunday, assess whether your pain level is better, the same, or worse. Do this for each of your symptoms, using a different-coloured pen for each symptom, week by week, creating a Progress Chart (an example is given on page 314). This system enables you to see what makes a difference. Make a note of which symptom is in which colour on your Progress Chart.

SETTING YOUR TARGETS

Be realistic in the targets you set. Take everything one step at a time. Set yourself targets that you know you will reach for changing your diet and taking exercise. It is far better to take one step towards permanently changing your lifestyle, than to take four steps back on an over-ambitious regime.

So, decide what you are going to do for the month ahead. Be realistic and specific; write it down and stick it up somewhere you can see it. This, plus weekly monitoring, will remind you to keep on track. Be patient with yourself. You can only make big changes to diet and lifestyle – which I believe are your best chances of conquering arthritis – by making a series of small, gradual changes. If you've had pain for five years, it may take you one year to find your ideal regime. The effects of exercise, diet and supplements are not as rapid as drugs, but they are cumulative. Once your diet and lifestyle have changed for the better, and you feel better, you will find you have little or no desire to go back to old habits.

RECORD CHANGES IN TREATMENT AND COMPLIANCE

Whenever you change your treatment, make a note of this. For example, if you decide to experiment with 1,000mg of B_3 (niacinamide) for a month, write this down. If your doctor lowers your medication dose, note this too. If you decide to avoid alcohol for a month, put this down as well. It is best not to make too many changes at once so that you can see which factor is making a difference.

At the end of each week rate yourself on your compliance with the targets you set yourself for diet, supplements and exercise (this could be physical exercise, hydrotherapy and/or postural exercises).

XXXX   means you met your targets. Well done.

XXX   means you more or less stuck to your targets. Good.

XX   means you only stuck to your targets half-heartedly.

X   means you went off the rails and didn't stick to your targets.

Notice what a difference your level of compliance makes to your health rating. Start every week afresh. If you didn't do well last week, that's history. This week, do your best to stick to your chosen goal.

On page 314 you'll see a sample of a complete Progress Chart over a 12-week period. Photocopy the blank Progress Chart on page 315, then write in the weeks and use this for the months that follow. Don't throw these charts away. Should you consult a health practitioner, the charts will help them to see, at a glance, how you've been getting on.

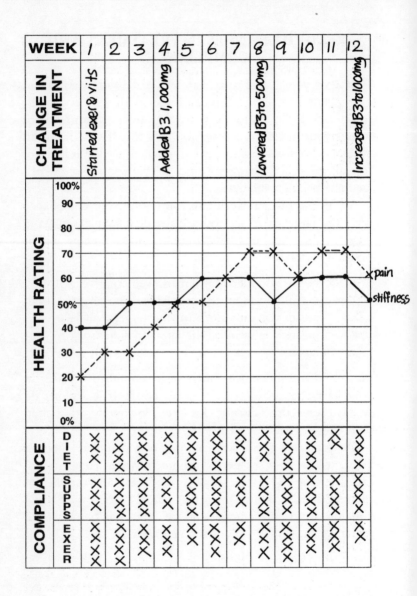

Figure 26 – Sample progress chart

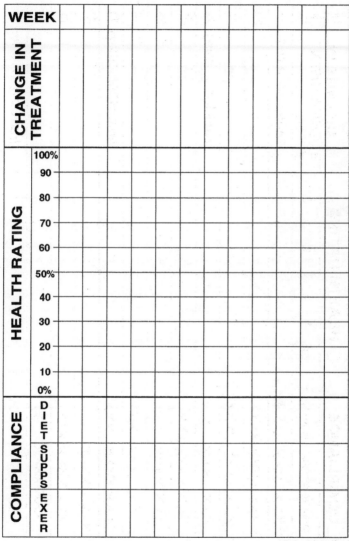

Figure 27 – Progress chart

REFERENCES

Part 1

1 J. H. Bland and S. M. Cooper, 'Osteoarthritis: A review of the cell biology involved and evidence for reversibility. Management rationally related to known genesis and pathophysiology', *Seminars in Arthritis and Rheumatism*, Vol 14(2) (1984), pp. 106–33

2 R. F. Meenan, et al., 'The impact of chronic disease: A sociomedical profile of rheumatoid arthritis', *Arthritis and Rheumatism*, Vol 24(3) (1981), pp. 544–9

3 Ellman and Mitchell in *Reports on Chronic Rheumatic Diseases*, ed., Buckley, Macmillan (1936)

4 E. K. Pradhan, et al., 'Effect of mindfulness-based stress reduction in rheumatoid arthritis patients', *Arthritis and Rheumatism*, Vol 57(7) (2007), pp. 1134–42

5 'Crime doesn't pay but keeps arthritis away', *Los Angeles Times*, 23 January 1963

6 J. C. Parker and B. D. Westra, 'Stress, psychological factors, and rheumatoid arthritis', *Current Opinion in Rheumatology*, Vol 1(1) (1989), pp. 39–43

7 D. Kiefe, 'Quenching the flames of inflammatory brain aging', *Life Extension Magazine* (September 2003)

8 J. J. Belch, et al., 'Effects of altering dietary essential fatty acids on requirements for non-steroidal anti-inflammatory drugs in patients with rheumatoid arthritis: A double blind placebo controlled study', *Annals of the Rheumatic Diseases*, Vol 47(2) (1988), pp. 96–104

9   J. M. Kremer, et al., 'Effects of manipulation of dietary fatty acids on clinical manifestations of rheumatoid arthritis', *Lancet*, Vol 1(8422) (1985), pp. 184–7; H. van der Tempel, et al., 'Effects of fish oil supplementation in rheumatoid arthritis', *Annals of the Rheumatic Diseases*, Vol 49(2) (1990), pp. 76–80; J. M. Kremer, et al., 'Dietary fish oil and olive oil supplementation in patients with rheumatoid arthritis: Clinical and immunologic effects', *Arthritis and Rheumatism*, Vol 33(6) (1990), pp. 810–20; G. L. Nielsen, et al., *European Journal of Clinical Investigation*, Vol 22 (1992), pp. 687–91; C. Jungeblut, 'Inactivation of poliomyelitis virus by crystalline vitamin C (ascorbic acid)', *Journal of Experimental Medicine*, Vol 62 (1935), pp. 517–21

10 C. Huerta, et al., 'Nonsteroidal anti-inflammatory drugs and risk of ARF in the general population', *American Journal of Kidney Diseases*, Vol 45(3) (2005), pp. 531–9

11 V. Kumar, et al., 'Robbins and Cotran pathologic basis of disease', pp. 1356–61, W.B. Saunders (1984). Petersdorf, et al., *Harrison's Principles of Internal Medicine*, McGraw Hill (1983), pp. 517–24

12 I. Bjarnason, et al., 'Intestinal permeability and inflammation in rheumatoid arthritis: Effects of non-steroidal anti-inflammatory drugs', *Lancet*, Vol 2(8413) (1984), pp. 1171–4

13 M. C. Allison, et al., 'Gastrointestinal damage associated with the use of nonsteroidal anti-inflammatory drugs', *New England Journal of Medicine*, Vol 327(11) (1992), pp. 749–54

14 Press release from American College of Rheumatology, 17 October 2004

15 M. M. Wolfe, et al., 'Gastrointestinal toxicity of non-steroidal anti-inflammatory drugs', *New England Journal of Medicine*, Vol 340(24) (1999), pp. 1888–99. This is for the years 1997 and 1998 and estimates 103,000 hospitalisations and 16,500 deaths each year

16 R. D. Rudic, et al., 'COX-2-derived prostacyclin modulates vascular remodelling', *Circulation Research*, Vol 96(12) (2005), pp. 1240–7

17 R. D. Rudic, et al., 'COX-2-derived prostacyclin modulates vascular remodelling', *Circulation Research*, Vol 96(12) (2005), pp. 1240–7

18 X. Liang, et al., 'Prostaglandin D2 mediates neuronal protection via the DP1 receptor', *Journal of Neurochemistry*, Vol 92(3) (2005), pp. 477–86. This essentially found that one of the effects of the prostaglandins blocked by COX-2 inhibitors was to protect brain

cells after a stroke. So, cutting down their production with the drug could increase stroke damage

19 C. Dai, et al., 'National trends in cyclooxygenase-2 inhibitor use since market release: Nonselective diffusion of a selectively cost-effective innovation', *Archives of Internal Medicine*, Vol 165(2) (2005), pp. 171–7

20 S. Chaplin, 'Volume and Cost of Prescribing in England (2004)', *Prescriber*, Vol 16(5) (5 August 2005). To print a hard copy, go to http://www.escriber.com/Prescriber/Features.asp?ID=989&GroupID=40&Action=View

21 J. Hippisley-Cox and C. Coupland, 'Risk of myocardial infarction in patients taking cyclo-oxygenase-2 inhibitors or conventional non-steroidal anti-inflammatory drugs: Population based nested case-control analysis', *British Medical Journal*, Vol 330(7504) (2005), pp. 1366–9

22 C. Huerta, et al., 'Non-steroidal anti-inflammatory drugs and risk of first hospital admission for heart failure in the general population', *Heart (British Cardiac Society)*, Vol 92(11) (2006), pp. 1610–15

23 P. Elwood, et al., 'For and against: Aspirin for everyone older than 50? For', *British Medical Journal*, Vol 330(7505) (2005), pp. 1440–1; C. Baigent, 'For and against: Aspirin for everyone older than 50? Against', *British Medical Journal*, Vol 330(7505) (2005), pp. 1442–3

24 'NSAIDs and adverse effects', See www.jr2.ox.ac.uk/bandolier/booth/painpag/nsae/nsae.html#Heading10

25 D. Y. Graham, et al., 'Visible small-intestinal mucosal injury in chronic NSAID users', *Clinical Gastroenterology and Hepatology*, Vol 3(1) (2005), pp. 55–9

26 P. M. Brooks, et al., 'NSAIDs and osteoarthritis: Help or hindrance?', *Journal of Rheumatology*, Vol 9(1) (1982), pp. 3–5

27 R. B. Raffa, et al., 'Discovery of "self-synergistic" spinal/supraspinal antinociception produced by acetaminophen (paracetamol)', *Journal of Pharmacology and Experimental Therapeutics*, Vol 295(1) (2000), pp. 291–4

28 Dr Anthony Temple, 'Max daily OTC dose of acetaminophen shows efficacy comparable to Rx doses of naproxen for OA pain', paper presented at the 2nd Joint Scientific Meeting of the American Pain Society and the Canadian Pain Society, 7 May 2004

29 T. E. Towheed, et al., 'Acetaminophen for osteoarthritis', *Cochrane Database of Systematic Reviews* (1): CD004257 (2006); T. Wienecke and P. C. Gøtzsche, 'Paracetamol versus nonsteroidal anti-inflammatory drugs for rheumatoid arthritis', *Cochrane Database of Systematic Reviews* (1): CD003789 (2004)

30 K. Hawton, et al., 'UK legislation on analgesic packs: Before and after study of long-term effect on poisonings', *British Medical Journal*, Vol 329(7474) (2004), p. 1076

31 L. Hunt, 'Ban pain drug, says leading surgeon', *Independent* (1 October 1996)

32 Youcha, 'The cortisone dilemma', *Science Digest* (January 1982)

33 L. M. Omland, et al., 'Risk factors for low bone mineral density among a large group of Norwegian women with fractures', *European Journal of Epidemiology*, Vol 16(3) (2000), pp. 223–9

34 J. M. Bjordal, et al., 'Non-steroidal anti-inflammatory drugs, including cyclo-oxygenase-2 inhibitors, in osteoarthritic knee pain: Meta-analysis of randomised placebo controlled trials', *British Medical Journal*, Vol 329(7478) (2004), p. 1317

35 G. Fitzgerald, 'Effect of ibuprofen on cardioprotective effect of aspirin', *Lancet*, Vol 361(9368) (2003), p. 1561

Part 2

1   N. Chainani-Wu, 'Safety and anti-inflammatory activity of curcumin: A Component of turmeric (curcuma longa)', *Journal of Alternative and Complementary Medicine*, Vol 9(1) (2003), pp. 161–8

2   B. Joe and B. R. Lokesh, 'Effect of curcumin and capsaicin on arachidonic acid metabolism and lysosomal enzyme secretion by rat peritoneal macrophages', *Lipids*, Vol 32(11) (1997), pp. 1173–80

3   G. C. Jagetia and B. B. Aggarwal, 'Spicing up of the immune system by curcumin', *Journal of Clinical Immunology*, Vol 27(1) (2007), pp. 19–35

4   A. Y. Fan, et al., 'Effects of an acetone extract of *Boswellia carterii Birdw.* (Burseraceae) gum resin on rats with persistent inflammation', *Journal of Alternative and Complementary Medicine*, Vol 11(2) (2005), pp. 323–31; A. Y. Fan, et al., 'Effects of an acetone extract of *Boswellia carterii Birdw.* (Burseraceae) gum resin on adjuvant-induced arthritis in Lewis rats', *Journal of Ethnopharmacology*, Vol 101(1–3) (2005), pp. 104–9

5   N. Kimmatkar, et al., 'Efficacy and tolerability of *Boswellia serrata* extract in treatment of osteoarthritis of knee: A randomized double-blind placebo controlled trial', *Phytomedicine*, Vol 10(1) (2003), pp. 3–7

6   V. Gupta, et al., 'Chemistry and pharmacology of gum resin of *Boswellia serrata*', *Indian Drugs*, Vol 24(5) (1986), pp. 221–31

7   H. Ichikawa, et al., 'Withanolides potentiate apoptosis, inhibit invasion, and abolish osteoclastogenesis through suppression of nuclear factor-kappaB (NF-kappaB) activation and NF-kappaB-regulated gene expression', *Molecular Cancer Therapeutics*, Vol 5(6) (2006), pp. 1434–45

8   R. R. Kulkarni, et al., 'Treatment of osteo-arthritis with a her-bomineral formulation: A double blind, placebo controlled, cross over study', *Journal of Ethnopharmacology*, Vol 33(1–2) (1991), pp. 91–5

9   M. Lindahl and C. Tagesson, 'Flavonoids as phospholipase A2 inhibitors: Importance of their structure for selective inhibition of group II phospholipase A2', *Inflammation*, Vol 21(3) (1997), pp. 347–56

10 Y. B. Shaik, et al., 'Role of quercetin (a natural herbal compound) in allergy and inflammation', *Journal of Biological Regulators and Homeostatic Agents*, Vol 20(3–4) (2006), pp. 47–52

11 A. Negre-Salvayre, et al., 'Additional antilipoperoxidant activities of alpha-tocopherol and ascorbic acid on membrane-like systems are potentiated by rutin', *Pharmacology*, Vol 42(5) (1991), pp. 262–72

12 F. Kiuchi, et al., 'Inhibition of prostaglandin and leukotriene biosynthesis by gingerols and diarylheptanoids', *Chemical and Pharmaceutical Bulletin*, Vol 40(2) (1992), pp. 387–91

13 B. H. Ali, et al., 'Some phytochemical, pharmacological and toxicological properties of ginger (*Zingiber officinale* Roscoe): A review of recent research', *Food and Chemical Toxicology*, Vol 46(2) (2008), pp. 409–20

14 K. C. Srivastava and T. Mustafa, 'Ginger (*Zingiber officianale*) and rheumatic disorders', *Medical Hypothesis*, Vol 39(4) (1992), pp. 342–8; R. D. Altman and K. C. Marcussen, 'Effects of a ginger extract on knee pain in patients with osteoarthitis', *Arthritis and Rheumatism*, Vol 44(11) (2001), pp. 2531–8

15 M. Lemay, et al., 'In vitro and ex vivo cyclooxygenase inhibition by a hops extract', *Asia Pacific Journal of Clinical Nutrition*, Vol 13 (supplement) (2004), p. S110

16 G. K. Beauchamp, et al., 'Phytochemistry: Ibuprofen-like activity in extra-virgin olive oil', *Nature*, Vol 437(7055) (2005), pp. 45–6

17 C. M. Bitler, et al., 'Hydrolyzed olive vegetation water in mice has anti-inflammatory activity', *Journal of Nutrition*, Vol 135(6) (2005), pp. 1475-9

18 R. C. Balagot, et al., 'Analgesia in mice and humans by D-phenyl-lalanine: Relation to inhibition of enkephalin degradation and enkephalin levels', in J. J. Bonica, J. C. Liebeskind and D. G. Albe-Fessard (eds.), *Advances in Pain Research and Therapy*, Vol 5, Raven Press (1983), pp. 289–93

19 K. Budd, 'Use of D-phenylalanine, an enkephalinase inhibitor, in the treatment of intractable pain', in J. J. Bonica, J. C. Liebeskind and D. G. Albe-Fessard (eds.), *Advances in Pain Research and Therapy*, Vol 5, Raven Press (1983), pp. 305–8

20 S. Ehrenpreis, et al., 'Naloxone reversible analgesia in mice produced by D-phenylalanine and hydrocinnamic acid, inhibitors of carboxypeptidase A', in J. J. Bonica, J. C. Liebeskind and D. G. Albe-Fessard (eds.), *Advances in Pain Research and Therapy*, Vol 3, Raven Press (1978), pp. 479–88

21 N. E. Walsh, et al., 'Analgesic effectiveness of D-phenylaline in chronic pain patients', *Archives of Physical Medicine and Rehabilitation*, Vol 67(7) (1986), pp. 436–9

22 Hopkins, *Anabolism*, Vol 4(2) (1985)

23 R. Widrig, et al., 'Choosing between NSAID and arnica for topical treatment of hand osteoarthritis in a randomised, double-blind study', *Rheumatology International*, Vol 27(6) (2007), pp. 585–91

24 O. Knuesel, et al., 'Arnica montana gel in osteoarthritis of the knee: An open, multicenter clinical trial', *Advances in Therapy*, Vol 19(5) (2002), pp. 209–18

25 W. J. Kraemer, et al., 'Effect of a cetylated fatty acid topical cream on functional mobility and quality of life of patients with osteoarthritis', *Journal of Rheumatology*, Vol 31(4) (2004), pp. 767–74

26 W. J. Kraemer, et al., 'Effects of treatment with a cetylated fatty acid topical cream on static postural stability and plantar pressure

distribution in patients with knee osteoarthritis', *Journal of Strength and Conditioning Research*, Vol 19(1) (2005), pp. 115–21

27 W. J. Kraemer, et al., 'A cetylated fatty acid topical cream with menthol reduces pain and improves functional performance in individuals with arthritis', *Journal of Strength and Conditioning Research*, Vol 19(2) (2005), pp. 475–80

28 C. L. Deal, et al., 'Treatment of arthritis with topical capsaicin: A double-blind trial', *Clinical Therapeutics*, Vol 13(3) (1991), pp. 383–95

29 G. M. McCarthy and D. J. McCarty, 'Effect of topical capsaicin in the therapy of painful osteoarthritis of the hands', *Journal of Rheumatology*, Vol 19(4) (1992), pp. 604–7

30 H. Frerick, et al., 'Topical treatment of chronic low back pain with a capsicum plaster', *Pain*, Vol 106(1–2) (2003), pp. 59–64; W. Keitel, et al., 'Capsicum pain plaster in chronic non-specific low back pain', *Arzneimittelforschung*, Vol 51(11) (2001), pp. 896–903

31 R. J. Goldberg, 'A meta-analysis of the analgesic effects of omega-3 polyunsaturated fatty acid supplementation for inflammatory joint pain', *Pain*, Vol 129(1–2) (2007), pp. 210–23

32 J. M. Kremer, et al., 'Effects of manipulation of dietary fatty acids on clinical manifestations of rheumatoid arthritis', *Lancet*, Vol 1(8422) (1985), pp. 184–7

33 H. van der Tempel, et al., 'Effects of fish oil supplementation in rheumatoid arthritis', *Annals of the Rheumatic Diseases*, Vol 49(2) (1990), pp. 76–80

34 J. M. Kremer, et al., 'Effects of manipulation of dietary fatty acids on clinical manifestations of rheumatoid arthritis', *Lancet*, Vol 325(8422) (1985), pp. 184–7; J. M. Kremer, et al., 'Dietary fish oil and olive oil supplementation in patients with rheumatoid arthritis: Clinical and immunologic effects', *Arthritis and Rheumatism*, Vol 33(6) (1990), pp. 810–20

35 G. L. Nielsen, et al., *European Journal of Clinical Investigation*, Vol 22 (1992), pp. 687–91

36 C. L. Curtis, et al., 'Pathologic indicators of degradation and inflammation in human osteoarthritic cartilage are abrogated by exposure to n-3 fatty acids', *Arthritis and Rheumatism*, Vol 46(6) (2002), pp. 1544–53

37 B. Galarraga, et al., 'Cod liver oil (n-3 fatty acids) as a non-steroidal

anti-inflammatory drug sparing agent in rheumatoid arthritis', *Rheumatology*, Vol 47(5) (2008), pp. 665–9

38 T. A. Mori, et al., 'Comparison of diets supplemented with fish oil or olive oil on plasma lipoproteins in insulin-dependent diabetics', *Metabolism*, Vol 40(3) (1991), pp. 241–6

39 G. Hansen, et al., 'Nutritional status of Danish patients with rheumatoid arthritis and effects of a diet adjusted in energy intake, fish content and antioxidants', *Ugeskrift for Laegeri*, Vol 160(21) (1998), pp. 3074–8

40 D. F. Horrobin, 'The regulation of prostaglandin biosynthesis: Negative feedback mechanisms and the selective control of formation of 1 and 2 series prostaglandins: Relevance to inflammation and immunity', *Medical Hypotheses*, Vol 6(7) (1980), pp. 687–709; R. B. Zurier and F. Quagliata, 'Effect of prostaglandin E 1 on adjuvant arthritis', *Nature*, Vol 234(5327) (1971), pp. 304–5; R. B. Zurier, et al., 'Prostaglandin E treatment of NZB/NZW mice', *Arthritis and Rheumatism*, Vol 20(2) (1977), pp. 723–8; S. L. Kunkel, et al., 'Species-dependent regulation of monocyte/macrophage Ia antigen expression and antigen presentation by prostaglandin E', *Cellular Immunology*, Vol 97(1) (1986), pp. 140–5

41 S. L. Kunkel, et al., 'Suppression of chronic inflammation by evening primrose oil', *Progress in Lipid Research*, Vol 20 (1981), pp. 885–8

42 R. A. Karmali, 'Effect of dietary fatty acids on experimental manifestation of Salmonella-associated arthritis in rats', *Prostaglandins, Leukotrienes and Medicine*, Vol 29(2–3) (1987), pp. 199–204

43 G. A. Tate, et al., 'Suppression of monosodium urate crystal-induced acute inflammation by diets enriched with gamma-linolenic acid and eicosapentaenoic acid', *Arthritis and Rheumatism*, Vol 31(12) (1988), pp. 1543–51

44 Hansen, et al., *Scandinavian Journal of Rheumatology*, Vol 6 (1989), pp. 729–33

45 J. M. Kremer, et al., 'Dietary fish oil and olive oil supplementation in patients with rheumatoid arthritis: Clinical and immunologic effects', *Arthritis and Rheumatism*, Vol 33(6) (1990), pp. 810–22

46 R. B. Zurier, et al., 'Gamma-linoleic acid treatment of rheumatoid arthritis: A randomised placebo-controlled trial', *Arthritis and Rheumatism*, Vol 39(11) (1996), pp. 1808–17

47 T. M. Hansen, et al., 'Treatment of rheumatoid arthritis with prostaglandin E1 precursors cis-linoleic acid and gamma-linolenic acid', *Scandinavian Journal of Rheumatology*,Vol 12(2) (1983), pp. 858

48 W. J. Kraemer, et al., 'Effect of a cetylated fatty acid topical cream on functional mobility and quality of life of patients with osteoarthritis', *Journal of Rheumatology*,Vol 31(4) (2004), pp. 767–74; R. Hesslink, et al.,'Cetylated fatty acids improve knee function in patients with osteoarthritis', *Journal of Rheumatology*, Vol 29(8) (2002), pp. 1708–12

49 R. Hesslink, et al.,'Cetylated fatty acids improve knee function in patients with osteoarthritis', *Journal of Rheumatology*, Vol 29(8) (2002), pp. 1708–12

50 J. H. Bland and S. M. Cooper, 'Osteoarthritis: A review of the cell biology involved and evidence for reversibility. Management rationally related to known genesis and pathophysiology', *Seminars in Arthritis and Rheumatism*,Vol 14(2) (1984), pp. 106–33

51 L. Sokoloff,'Endemic forms of osteoarthritis', *Clinics in Rheumatic Diseases*,Vol 11(2) (1985), pp. 187–202

52 Kroker, et al., Clin. Ecol.,Vol 2 (1984), pp. 137–44; A. M. Uden, et al.,'Neutrophil functions and clinical performance after total fasting in patients with rheumatoid arthritis', *Annals of the Rheumatic Diseases*,Vol 42(1) (1983), pp. 45–51; T. Sundqvist, et al., 'Influence of fasting on intestinal permeability and disease activity in patients with rheumatoid arthritis', *Scandinavian Journal of Rheumatology*,Vol 11(1) (1982), pp. 33–8

53 L. G. Darlington,'Dietary therapy for arthritis', *Rheumatic Diseases Clinics of North America*,Vol 17(2) (1991), pp. 273–85

54 S. N. Lichtman, et al., 'Reactivation of arthritis induced by small bowel bacterial overgrowth in rats: Role of cytokines, bacteria, and bacterial polymers', *Infection and Immunity*, Vol 63(6) (1995), pp. 2295–301

55 M. P. Hazenberg, 'Intestinal flora bacteria and arthritis: Why the joint?' *Scandinavian Journal of Rheumatology*, 101 (Supplement) (1995), pp. 207–11; J. O. Hunter, 'Food allergy or enterometabolic disorder?' *Lancet*,Vol 338(8765) (1991), pp. 495–6

56 I. Bjarnason, et al., 'Intestinal permeability and inflammation in rheumatoid arthritis: Effects of non-steroidal anti-inflammatory drugs', *Lancet*, Vol 2(8413) (1984), pp. 1171–4; H. Mielants,

'Reflections on the link between intestinal permeability and inflammatory joint disease', *Clinical and Experimental Rheumatology*, Vol 8(5) (1990), pp. 523–4

57 H. Bradley, et al., 'Metabolism of low-dose paracetamol in patients with rheumatoid arthritis', *Xenobiotica*, Vol 21(5) (1991), pp. 689–93

58 Royal College of Physicians report, *Allergy: Conventional and Alternative Concepts* (1992)

59 M. A. van der Laar and J. K. van der Korst, 'Food intolerance in rheumatoid arthritis: I. A double blind, controlled trial of the clinical effects of elimination of milk allergens and azo dyes', *Annals of Rheumatic Diseases*, Vol 51(3) (1992), pp. 298–302; M. A. van der Laar and J. K. van der Korst, 'Food intolerance in rheumatoid arthritis: II. Clinical and histological aspects', *Annals of Rheumatic Diseases*, Vol 51(3) (1992), pp. 303–6

60 T. Jalonen, 'Identical intestinal permeability changes in children with different clinical manifestations of cow's milk allergy', *Journal of Allergy and Clinical Immunology*, Vol 88(5) (1991), pp. 737–42; see also N. Kalach, et al., 'Intestinal permeability in children: Variation with age and reliability in the diagnosis of cow's milk allergy', *Acta Paediatrica*, Vol 90(5) (2001), pp. 499–504

61 J. A. Hicklin, et al., 'The effect of diet in rheumatoid arthritis', *Clinical Allergy*, Vol 10(4) (1980), p. 463

62 C. O'Farrelly, et al., 'Association between villous atrophy in rheumatoid arthritis and a rheumatoid factor and gliadin-specific IgG', *Lancet*, Vol 2(8615) (1988), pp. 819–22

63 R. S. Panush, et al., 'Food-induced (allergic) arthritis. Inflammatory arthritis exacerbated by milk', *Arthritis and Rheumatism*, Vol 29(2) (1986), pp. 220–6

64 D. Ratner, et al., 'Juvenile rheumatoid arthritis and milk allergy', *Journal of the Royal Society of Medicine*, Vol 78(5) (1985), pp. 410–13; A. L. Parke and G. R. Hughes, 'Rheumatoid arthritis and food: A case study', *British Medical Journal*, Vol 282(6281) (1981), pp. 2027–9

65 Marshall, et al., Clin. Ecol., Vol 2 (1984), pp. 180–90

66 T. Sundqvist, et al., 'Influence of fasting on intestinal permeability and disease activity in patients with rheumatoid arthritis', *Scandinavian Journal of Rheumatology*, Vol 11(1) (1982), pp. 33–8

67 L. Skoldstam, 'Fasting and vegan diet in rheumatoid arthritis', *Scandinavian Journal of Rheumatology*, Vol 15(2) (1986), pp. 219–23

68 J. Kjeldsen-Kragh, et al., 'Controlled trial of fasting and one-year vegetarian diet in rheumatoid arthritis', *Lancet*, Vol 338(8772) (1991), pp. 899–902

69 N. F. Childers and G. M. Russo, *The Nightshades and Health*, Horticulture Publications, Somerville (1977)

70 A. Zampelas, et al., 'Association between coffee consumption and inflammatory markers in healthy persons: The ATTICA study', *American Journal of Clinical Nutrition*, Vol 80(4) (2004), pp. 862–7; A 50 per cent higher level of one of the markers (known as interleukin 6), a 30 per cent higher level of another (known as C-reactive protein) and a 28 per cent higher level of a third (known as TNF) compared to non-coffee consumers

71 D. J. Pattison, et al., 'Dietary beta-cryptoxanthin and inflammatory polyarthritis: Results from a population-based prospective study', *American Journal of Clinical Nutrition*, Vol 82(2) (2005), pp. 451–5

72 J. I. Rodale, *The Complete Book of Vitamins*, Rodale Press (1977)

73 M. Yazar, et al., 'Synovial fluid and plasma selenium, copper, zinc, and iron concentrations in patients with rheumatoid arthritis and osteoarthritis', *Biological Trace Element Research*, Vol 106(2) (2005), pp. 123–32; N. Ahmadzadeh, et al., 'Iron-binding proteins and free iron in synovial fluids of rheumatoid arthritis patients', *Clinical Rheumatology*, Vol 8(3) (1989), pp. 345–51; P. Biemond, et al., 'Intraarticular ferritin-bound iron in rheumatoid arthritis: A factor that increases oxygen free radical-induced tissue destruction', *Arthritis and Rheumatism*, Vol 29(10) (1986), pp. 1187–93

74 Conference presentation: Blake, 'Iron overload in rheumatoid arthritis', Brain Bio Center, New Jersey, USA (1981)

75 D. A. Rowley and B. Halliwell, 'Formation of hydroxyl radicals from hydrogen peroxide and iron salts by superoxide- and ascorbate-dependent mechanisms: Relevance to the pathology of rheumatoid disease', *Clinical Science (London)*, Vol 64(6) (1983), pp. 649–53

76 W. Niedermeier and J. H. Griggs, 'Trace metal composition of synovial fluid and blood serum of patients with rheumatoid arthritis', *Journal of Chronic Diseases*, Vol 23(8) (1971), pp. 527–36; S. P. Pandey, et al., 'Zinc in rheumatoid arthritis', *Indian Journal of Medical Research*, Vol 81 (1985), pp. 618–20; K. L. Svenson, et al.,

'Reduced zinc in peripheral blood cells from patients with inflammatory connective tissue diseases', *Inflammation*, Vol 9(2) (1985), pp. 189–99

77 P. A. Simpkin, 'Oral zinc sulphate in rheumatoid arthritis', *Lancet*, Vol 2(7985) (1976), pp. 539–42

78 O. J. Clemmensen, et al., 'Psoriatic arthritis treated with oral zinc sulphate', *British Journal of Dermatology*, Vol 103(4) (1980), pp. 411–15

79 J. J. Rasker and S. H. Kardaun, 'Lack of beneficial effect of zinc sulphate in rheumatoid arthritis', *Scandinavian Journal of Rheumatology*, Vol 11(3) (1982), pp. 168–70

80 Bland, *Int. Clin. Nutrition Rev.*, Vol 4(3) (1984), pp. 130–4

81 W. Niedermeier, 'Concentration and chemical state of copper in synovial fluid and blood serum of patients with rheumatoid arthritis', *Annals of the Rheumatic Diseases*, Vol 24(6), 1965, pp. 544–8; W. Niedermeier and J. H. Griggs, 'Trace metal composition of synovial fluid and blood serum of patients with rheumatoid arthritis', *Journal of Chronic Diseases*, Vol 23(8) (1971), pp. 527–36

82 W. R. Walker and D. M. Keats, 'An investigation of the therapeutic value of the "copper bracelet": Dermal assimilation of copper in arthritic/rheumatoid conditions', *Agents & Actions*, Vol 6(4) (1976), pp. 454–9

83 R. J. Shamberger, 'Relationship of selenium to cancer: I. Inhibitory effect of selenium on carcinogenesis', *Journal of the National Cancer Institute*, Vol 44(4) (1970), pp. 931–6; R. J. Shamberger, et al., 'Antioxidants and cancer: I. Selenium in the blood of normals and cancer patients', *Journal of the National Cancer Institute*, Vol 50(4), 1973, pp. 863–70; G. N. Schrauzer and D. Ishmael, 'Effects of selenium and of arsenic on the genesis of spontaneous mammary tumors in inbred C3H mice', *Annals of Clinical and Laboratory Science*, Vol 4(6) (1974), pp. 441–7; W. C. Willett, et al., 'Prediagnostic serum selenium and risk of cancer', *Lancet*, Vol 2(8342) (1983), pp. 130–4

84 K. Kose, et al., 'Plasma selenium levels in rheumatoid arthritis', *Biological Trace Element Research*, Vol 53(1–3) (1996), pp. 51–6; U. Johansson, et al., 'Nutritional status in girls with juvenile chronic arthritis', *Human Nutrition, Clinical Nutrition*, Vol 40(1) (1986), pp.

57–67; U. Tarp, et al., 'Low selenium level in severe rheumatoid arthritis', *Scandinavian Journal of Rheumatology*, Vol 14(2) (1985), pp. 97–101; J. Aaseth, et al., 'Trace elements in serum and urine of patients with rheumatoid arthritis', *Scandinavian Journal of Rheumatology*, Vol 7(4) (1978), pp. 237–40

85 A. Peretz, et al., 'Adjuvant treatment of recent onset rheumatoid arthritis by selenium supplementation: Preliminary observations', *British Journal of Rheumatology*, Vol 31(4) (1992), pp. 281–2

86 K. Heinle, et al., 'Selenium concentration in erythrocytes of patients with rheumatoid arthritis: Clinical and laboratory chemistry infection markers during administration of selenium', *Medizinische Klinik*, Vol 92 (supplement 3) (1997), pp. 29–31

87 P. Roberts, et al., 'Vitamin C and inflammation', *Medical Biology*, Vol 62(2) (1984), p. 88

88 E. R. Schwartz, 'The modulation of osteoarthritic development by vitamins C and E', *International Journal for Vitamin and Nutrition Research* (Supplement), Vol 26 (1984), pp. 141–6

89 J. Greenwood Jr., 'Optimum vitamin C intake as a factor in the preservation of disc integrity: Preliminary report', *The Medical Annals of the District of Columbia*, Vol 33, 1964, pp. 274–6

90 S. Goodman, *Vitamin C: The Master Nutrient*, Keats (1992)

91 Yoshikawa, et al., 'Studies on the pathogenesis of rheumatoid arthritis: I. lipid peroxide and lysosomal enzymes in rheumatoid joints', *Japanese Journal of Medicine*, Vol 18(3) (1979), pp. 199–204

92 Machtey and Ouaknine, *Journal of the American Geriatrics Society*, Vol 26(7) (1979), pp. 328–30

93 T. Yoshikawa, et al., 'Effect of vitamin E on adjuvant arthritis in rats', *Biochemical Medicine*, Vol 29(2) (1983), pp. 227–34

94 S. E. Edmonds, et al., 'Putative analgesic activity of repeated oral doses of vitamin E in the treatment of rheumatoid arthritis: Results of a prospective placebo controlled double blind trial', *Annals of the Rheumatic Diseases*, Vol 56(11) (1997), pp. 649–55

95 B. Kowsari, et al., 'Assessment of the diet of patients with rheumatoid arthritis and osteoarthritis', *Journal of the American Dietetic Association*, Vol 82(6) (1983), pp. 657–9

96 O. Hänninen, et al., 'Antioxidants in vegan diet and rheumatic disorders', *Toxicology*, Vol 155(1–3) (2000), pp. 45–53

97   C. T. Nelson, et al., 'Changes in endochondral ossification of the tibia accompanying acute pantothenic acid deficiency in young rats', *Proceedings of the Society of Experimental Biology and Medicine*, Vol 73(1) (1950), pp. 31–6

98   J. C. Annand, 'Pantothenic acid and osteoarthritis', *Lancet*, Vol 2(7318) (1963), p. 1168

99   E. C. Barton-Wright and W. A. Elliott, 'The pantothenic acid metabolism of rheumatoid arthritis', *Lancet*, Vol 2(7313) (1963), pp. 862–3

100 No authors listed, 'Calcium pantothenate in arthritic conditions: A report from the General Practitioner Research Group', *Practitioner*, Vol 224(1340) (1980), pp. 208–11

101 A. Hoffer, 'Treatment of arthritis by nicotinic acid and nicotinamide', *Canadian Medical Association Journal*, Vol 81 (1959), pp. 235–8

102 W. Kaufman, 'The use of vitamin therapy to reverse certain concomitants of aging', *Journal of the American Geriatrics Society*, Vol 3(11), 1955, pp. 927–36

103 W. B. Jonas, et al., 'The effect of niacinamide on osteoarthritis: A pilot study', *Inflammation Research*, Vol 45(7) (1996), pp. 330–4

104 S. G. Chrysant and M. Ibrahim, 'Niacin-ER/statin combination for the treatment of dyslipidemia: Focus on low high-density lipoprotein cholesterol', *Journal of Clinical Hypertension (Greenwich, Conn.)*, Vol 8(7) (2006), pp. 493–9; M. Miller, 'Niacin as a component of combination therapy for dyslipidemia', *Mayo Clinic Proceedings*, Vol 78(6) (2003), pp. 735–42

105 L. R. Mosher, 'Nicotinic acid side effects and toxicity: A review', *The American Journal of Psychiatry*, Vol 126(9) (1970), pp. 1290–6

106 J. M. Ellis, *Free of Pain: A Proven and Inexpensive Treatment for Specific Types of Rheumatism*, Southwest Publishing (1983)

107 J. M. Ellis, et al., 'Response of vitamin B-6 deficiency and the carpal tunnel syndrome to pyridoxine', *Proceedings of the National Academy of Sciences USA*, Vol 79(23) (1982), pp. 7494–8

108 M. A. Flynn, et al., 'The effect of folate and cobalamin on osteoarthritic hands', *Journal of the American College of Nutrition*, Vol 13(4) (1994), pp. 351–6

109 M. G. Signorello, et al., 'Effect of homocysteine on arachidonic acid release in human platelets', *European Journal of Clinical Investigation*, Vol 32(4) (2002), pp. 279–84

110 R. Roubenoff, et al., 'Abnormal homocysteine metabolism in rheumatoid arthritis', *Arthritis and Rheumatism*, Vol 40(4) (1997), pp. 718–22

111 K. Woolf and M. M. Manore, 'Elevated plasma homocysteine and low vitamin B-6 status in nonsupplementing older women with rheumatoid arthritis', *Journal of the American Dietetic Association*, Vol 108(3) (2008), pp. 443–53

112 A. Hernanz, et al., 'Increased plasma levels of homocysteine and other thiol compounds in rheumatoid arthritis women', *Clinical Biochemistry*, Vol 32(1) (1999), pp. 65–70

113 B. Seriolo, et al., 'Homocysteine and antiphospholipid antibodies in rheumatoid arthritis patients: Relationships with thrombotic events', *Clinical and Experimental Rheumatology*, Vol 19(5) (2001), pp. 561–4

114 X. M. Gao, et al., 'Homocysteine, ankylosing spondylitis and reactive arthritis: Homocysteine modification of HLA antigens and its immunological consequences', *European Journal of Immunology*, Vol 26(7) (1996), pp. 1443–50

115 P. E. Lazzerini, et al., 'Homocysteine enhances cytokine production in cultured synoviocytes from rheumatoid arthritis patients', *Clinical and Experimental Rheumatology*, Vol 24(4) (2006), pp. 387–93

116 M. A. Flynn, et al., 'The effect of folate and cobalamin on osteoarthritic hands', *Journal of the American College of Nutrition*, Vol 13(4), 1994, pp. 351–6

117 J. M. Ellis, *Free of Pain: A Proven Inexpensive Treatment for Specific Types of Rheumatism*, Southwest Publishing (1983)

118 C. Desouza, et al., 'Drugs affecting homocysteine metabolism: Impact on cardiovascular risk', *Drugs*, Vol 62(4) (2002), pp. 605–16; R. Fijnheer, et al., 'Homocysteine, methylenetetrahydrofolate reductase polymorphism, antiphospholipid antibodies, and thromboembolic events in systemic lupus erythematosus: A retrospective cohort study', *Journal of Rheumatology*, Vol 25(9) (1998), pp. 1737–42

119 R. Fijnheer, et al., 'Homocysteine, methylenetetrahydrofolate reductase polymorphism, antiphospholipid antibodies, and thromboembolic events in systemic lupus erythematosus: A retrospective cohort study', *Journal of Rheumatology*, Vol 25(9) (1998), pp. 1737–42

120 M. Krogh Jensen, et al., 'Folate and homocysteine status and haemolysis in patients treated with sulphasalazine for arthritis', *Scandinavian Journal of Clinical Laboratory Investigation*, Vol 56(5) (1996), pp. 421–9

121 A. E. van Ede, et al., 'Homocysteine and folate status in methotrexate-treated patients with rheumatoid arthritis', *Rheumatology (Oxford)*, Vol 41(6) (2002), pp. 658–65; O. Slot, 'Changes in plasma homocysteine in arthritis patients starting treatment with low-dose methotrexate subsequently supplemented with folic acid', *Scandinavian Journal of Rheumatology*, Vol 30(5) (2001), pp. 305–7; N. Hornung, et al., 'Folate, homocysteine, and cobalamin status in patients with rheumatoid arthritis treated with methotrexate, and the effect of low dose folic acid supplement', *Journal of Rheumatology*, Vol 31(12) (2004), pp. 2374–81; M. Hoekstra, et al., 'Intermittent rises in plasma homocysteine in patients with rheumatoid arthritis treated with higher dose methotrexate', *Annals of the Rheumatic Diseases*, Vol 64(1) (2005), pp. 141–3; C. J. Haagsma, et al., 'Influence of sulphasalazine, methotrexate, and the combination of both on plasma homocysteine concentrations in patients with rheumatoid arthritis', *Annals of the Rheumatic Diseases*, Vol 58(2) (1999), pp. 79–84

122 K. Koyama, et al., 'Efficacy of methylcobalamin on lowering total homocysteine plasma concentrations in haemodialysis patients receiving high-dose folate supplementation', *Nephrology Dialysis Transplantation*, Vol 17(5) (2002), pp. 916–22

123 G. M. Hall, et al., 'Depressed levels of dehydroepiandrosterone sulphate in postmenopausal women with rheumatoid arthritis but no relation with axial bone density', *Annals of the Rheumatic Diseases*, Vol 52(3) (1993), pp. 211–14

124 J. Pizzorno and M. Murray (eds.), *The Textbook of Natural Medicine*, John Bastyr College (1987)

125 Ibid.

Part 3

1 NASA report, American Medical Association Symposium, Florida (1982); M. Korcak, *Journal of the American Medical Association*, Vol 247 (1982), p. 8

2 J. R. Marier, 'Magnesium content of the food supply in the modern-day world', *Magnesium*, Vol 5(1) (1986), pp. 1–8

3   J. L. Loughead, et al., 'A role for magnesium in neonatal parathy-
     roid gland function', *Journal of the American College of Nutrition*, Vol
     10(2) (1991), pp. 123–6

4   Hamilton & Minski, *Sci. Total Environ.*, Vol 1, 1972/3, p. 375

5   G. E. Abraham, 'The importance of magnesium in the manage-
     ment of primary postmenopausal osteoporosis', *Journal of Nutri-
     tional Medicine*, Vol 2(2) (1991), pp. 165–78

6   Z. Andjelkovic, et al., 'Disease modifying and immunomodulatory
     effects of high dose 1 alpha (OH) D3 in rheumatoid arthritis patients',
     Clinical and Experimental Rheumatology, Vol 17(4) (1999), pp. 453-61; J.
     Brohult and B. Jonson, 'Effects of large doses of calciferol on patients
     with rheumatoid arthritis: A double-blind clinical trial', *Scandinavian
     Journal of Rheumatology*, Vol 2(4) (1973), pp. 173–6 (reduced disease
     activity); L. Dottori, et al., 'Calcifediol and calcitonin in the therapy of
     rheumatoid arthritis. A short-term controlled study', *Minerva Medica*,
     Vol 73(43) (1982), pp. 3033–40 (pain reduction)

7   A. Zittermann, 'Vitamin D in preventive medicine: Are we ignor-
     ing the evidence?' *British Journal of Nutrition*, Vol 89(5) (2003), pp.
     552–72

8   B. Lamke, et al., 'Bone mineral content in women with vertebral
     fractures', *Acta Medica Scandinavica*, Vol 207(1–2) (1980), pp. 71–2;
     C. J. Lee, et al., 'Effects of supplementation of the diets with cal-
     cium and calcium-rich foods on bone density of elderly females
     with osteoporosis', *American Journal of Clinical Nutrition*, Vol 34(5),
     (1981), pp. 819–23; E. L. Smith Jr., et al., 'Physical activity and cal-
     cium modalities for bone mineral increase in aged women', *Medi-
     cine and Science in Sports and Exercise*, Vol 13(1), (1981), pp. 60–4

9   M. W. Tilyard, et al., 'Treatment of postmenopausal osteoporosis
     with calcitriol or calcium', *New England Journal of Medicine*, Vol
     326(6) (1992), pp. 57–62

10   M. K. Thomas, et al., 'Hypovitaminosis D in medical inpatients',
     New England Journal of Medicine, Vol 338(12) (1998), pp. 777–83

11   C. Simonelli, et al., 'Prevalence of vitamin D inadequacy in a min-
     imal trauma fracture population', *Current Medical Research Opinion*,
     Vol 21(7) (2005), pp. 1069–74

12   S. Gaugris, et al., 'Vitamin D inadequacy among post-menopausal
     women: A systematic review', *Quarterly Journal of Medicine*, Vol
     98(9) (2005), pp. 667–76

13 R. Vieth, et al., 'The urgent need to recommend an intake of vita-
    min D that is effective', *American Journal of Clinical Nutrition*, Vol
    85(3) (2007), pp. 649–50

14 M. F. Holick, 'Michael Holick, PhD, MD: Vitamin D pioneer.
    Interview by Frank Lampe and Suzanne Snyder', *Alternative Ther-
    apies in Health and Medicine*, Vol 14(3) (2008), pp. 65–75

15 G. A. Plotnikoff and J. M. Quigley, 'Prevalence of severe hypovita-
    minosis D in patients with persistent, nonspecific musculoskeletal
    pain', *Mayo Clinic Proceedings*, Vol 78(12) (2003), pp. 1463–70

16 F. S. Al and M. K. Al, 'Vitamin D deficiency and chronic low back
    pain in Saudi Arabia', *Spine*, Vol 28(2) (2003), pp. 177–9

17 M. F. Holick, 'Vitamin D: Importance in the prevention of cancers,
    type 1 diabetes, heart disease, and osteoporosis', *American Journal of
    Clinical Nutrition*, Vol 79(3) (2004), pp. 362–71

18 F. H. Nielsen, 'Is boron nutritionally relevant?' *Nutrition Reviews*,
    Vol 66(4) (2008), pp. 183–91

19 R. E. Newnham, 'Mineral imbalance and boron deficiency', in
    Trace Element Metabolism in Man and Animals (Tema-4), Australian
    Academy of Science (1981), pp. 400–2; and 'Boron is Essential: It
    Corrects and Prevents Arthritis', conference presentation of the
    New Zealand Trace Element Group, Massey University, New
    Zealand (7–8 August 1984)

20 N. Ward, *Journal of Radioanalytical and Nuclear Chemistry, Articles*,
    Vol 110(2) (1987), p. 633

21 F. H. Neilson, et al., 'Effect of dietary boron on mineral, estrogen,
    and testosterone metabolism in postmenopausal women', *The
    FASEB Journal*, Vol 1(5) (1987), pp. 394–7

22 R. L. Travers, et al., 'Boron and arthritis: The results of a double-
    blind pilot study', *Journal of Nutritional Medicine*, Vol 1 (1990), pp.
    127–32

23 O. Gillie, 'Sunlight, Vitamin D & Health: A report of a conference
    held at the House of Commons in November 2005', Health
    Research Forum Occasional Reports: No. 2 (Full Report can be
    downloaded at http://www.healthresearchforum.org.uk/reports/
    sunbook.pdf).

24 Mankin, *Orthopedic Clinics of North America*, Vol 2 (1972), p. 19

25 I. Setnikar, et al., 'Pharmacokinetics of glucosamine in the dog and
    in man', *Arzneimittel-Forschung*, Vol 36(4) (1986), pp. 729–35

26 K. Karzel and K. J. Lee, 'Effect of hexosamine derivatives on mesenchymal metabolic processes of in vitro cultured fetal bone explants', *Zeitschrift fur Rheumatologie*, Vol 41(5) (1982), pp. 212–18; I. Setnikar, et al., 'Antireactive properties of glucosamine sulfate', *Arzneimittel-Forschung*, Vol 41(2) (1991), pp. 157–61

27 M. T. Muraty, 'Glucosamine sulfate: Effective osteoarthritis treatment', *American Journal of Natural Medicine* (10–14 September 1994)

28 J. Y. Reginster, et al., 'Long-term effects of glucosamine sulphate on osteoarthritis progression: A randomised, placebo-controlled clinical trial', *Lancet*, Vol 357(9252) (2001), pp. 251–6

29 G. X. Qui, et al., 'Efficacy and safety of glucosamine sulfate versus ibuprofen in patients with knee osteoarthritis', *Arzneimittel-Forschung*, Vol 48(5) (1998), pp. 469–74

30 T. E. Towheed, et al., 'Glucosamine therapy for treating osteoarthritis', *The Cochrane Database of Systematic Reviews* (2): CD002946 (2005)

31 H. J. Hehne, et al., 'Therapy of gonarthrosis using chondroprotective substances: Prospective comparative study of glucosamine sulphate and glycosaminoglycan polysulphate', *Fortschritte der Medizin*, Vol 102(24) (1984), pp. 676–82

32 A. Lopes Vaz, 'Double-blind clinical evaluation of the relative efficacy of ibuprofen and glucosamine sulphate in the management of osteoarthrosis of the knee in out-patients', *Current Medical Research and Opinion*, Vol 8(3) (1982), pp. 145–9

33 D. O. Clegg, et al., 'Glucosamine, Chondroitin Sulfate, and the two in combination for painful knee osteoarthritis', *New England Journal of Medicine*, Vol 354(8) (2006), pp. 795–808

34 D. O. Clegg, et al., 'Glucosamine, Chondroitin Sulfate, and the two in combination for painful knee osteoarthritis', *New England Journal of Medicine*, Vol 354(8) (2006), pp. 795–808

35 B. Mazieres, et al., 'Chondroitin sulfate in osteoarthritis of the knee: A prospective, double blind, placebo controlled multicenter clinical study', *Journal of Rheumatology*, Vol 28(1) (2001), pp. 173–81; F. Richy, et al., 'Structural and symptomatic efficacy of glucosamine and chondroitin in knee osteoarthritis: A comprehensive meta-analysis', *Archives of Internal Medicine*, Vol 163(13) (2003), pp. 1514–22

36 B. C. Jang, et al., 'Glucosamine hydrochloride specifically inhibits COX-2 by preventing COX-2 N-glycosylation and by increasing COX-2 protein turnover in a proteasome-dependent manner', *Journal of Biological Chemistry*, Vol 282(38) (2007), pp. 27622–32

37 Methylsulfonylmethane (MSM) Monograph, *Alternative Medicine Review*, Vol 8(4) (2003), pp. 438–41

38 S. W. Jacob MD, R. M. Lawrence MD PhD and M. Zucker, *The Miracle of MSM: The Natural Solution for Pain*, Putnam (1999).

39 S. W. Jacob and J. Appleton, *MSM: The Definitive Guide. A Comprehensive Review of the Science and Therapeutics of Methylsulfonylmethane*, Freedom Press (2003), pp. 107–121

40 P. R. Usha and M. U. Naidu, 'Randomised, double-blind, parallel, placebo-controlled study of oral glucosamine, methylsulfonylmethane and their combination in osteoarthritis', *Clinical Drug Investigation*, Vol 24(6) (2004), pp. 353–63

41 S. W. Jacob and J. Appleton, *MSM: The Definitive Guide. A Comprehensive Review of the Science and Therapeutics of Methylsulfonylmethane*, Freedom Press (2003), pp. 107–21

42 R. G. Gibson, et al., 'Perna canaliculus in the treatment of arthritis', *The Practitioner*, Vol 224(1347) (1980), pp. 955–60

43 A. F. El-Ghobarey, et al., 'Clinical and laboratory studies of levamisole in patients with rheumatoid arthritis', *Quarterly Journal of Medicine*, Vol 47(187) (1978), pp. 385–400

44 L. Solomon, 'Drug-induced arthropathy and necrosis of the femoral head', *Journal of Bone and Joint Surgery*, Vol 55(2) (1973), pp. 246–61

45 R. Marcolongo, et al., 'Double-blind multicentre study of the activity of S-adenosyl-methionine in hip and knee osteoarthritis', *Current Therapeutic Research, Clinical and Experimental*, Vol 37 (1985), pp. 82–94

46 J. D. Bradley, et al., 'A randomized, double blind, placebo controlled trial of intravenous loading with S-adenosylmethionine (SAM) followed by oral SAM therapy in patients with knee osteoarthritis', *Journal of Rheumatology*, Vol 21(5), 1994, pp. 905–11

47 E. Cameron and L. Pauling, 'Supplemental ascorbate in the supportive treatment of cancer: Prolongation of survival times in terminal human cancer', *Proceedings of the National Academy of Sciences*,

Vol 73(10) (1976), pp. 3685–9; E. Cameron and L. Pauling, 'Supplemental ascorbate in the supportive treatment of cancer: Reevaluation of prolongation of survival times in terminal human cancer', *Proceedings of the National Academy of Sciences*, Vol 75(9) (1978), pp. 4538–42

48 M. Colgan, *Your Personal Vitamin Profile*, Blond & Briggs (1983)

Part 4

1   G. F. Gordon, 'New dimensions in calcium metabolism', *Osteopathic Annals* (1983)

2   Morter, Correlative Urinalysis, BEST Research Inc (1987); R. B. Mazess and W. Mather, 'Bone mineral content in North Alaskan Eskimos', *American Journal of Clinical Nutrition*, Vol 27(9) (1974), pp. 916–25

3   D. Feskanich, et al., 'Protein consumption and bone fractures in women', *American Journal of Epidemiology*, Vol 143(5) (1996), pp. 472–9

4   L. H. Allen, et al., 'Protein-induced hypercalcuria: A longer-term study', *American Journal of Clinical Nutrition*, Vol 32(4) (1979), pp. 741–9; C. R. Anand and H. M. Linkswiler, 'Effect of protein intake on calcium balance of young men given 500mg calcium daily', *Journal of Nutrition*, Vol 104(6) (1974), pp. 695–700

5   R. G. Cumming, et al., 'Calcium intake and fracture risk: Results from the study of osteoporotic fractures', *American Journal of Epidemiology*, Vol 145(10) (1997), pp. 926–34

6   S. T. Reddy, et al., 'Effect of low-carbohydrate high-protein diets on acid-base balance, stone-forming propensity, and calcium metabolism', *American Journal of Kidney Diseases*, Vol 40(2) (2002), pp. 265–74

7   L. H. Allen, et al., 'Protein-induced hypercalciuria: A longer term study', *American Journal of Clinical Nutrition*, Vol 32(4) (1979), pp. 741–9

8   A. Wachman and D. S. Bernstein, 'Diet and osteoporosis', *Lancet*, Vol 1(7549), 1968, pp. 958–9

9   D. Feskanich, et al., 'Milk, dietary calcium, and bone fractures in women: A 12-year prospective study', *American Journal of Public Health*, Vol 97(6) (1997), pp. 992–7

10 M. Miyao, et al., 'Association of methylenetetrahydrofolate

reductase (MTHFR) polymorphism with bone mineral density in postmenopausal Japanese women', *Calcified Tissue International*, Vol 66(3) (2000), pp. 190–4

11 C. G. Gjesdal, et al., 'Plasma total homocysteine level and bone mineral density: The Hordaland Homocysteine Study', *Archives of Internal Medicine*, Vol 166(1) (2006), pp. 88–94; R. R. McLean, et al., 'Homocysteine as a predictive factor for hip fracture in older persons', *New England Journal of Medicine*, Vol 350(20) (2004), pp. 2042–9; J. B. van Meurs, et al., 'Homocysteine levels and the risk of osteoporotic fracture', *New England Journal of Medicine*, Vol 350(20) (2004), pp. 2033–41

12 C. G. Gjesdal, et al., 'Plasma homocysteine, folate, and vitamin B 12 and the risk of hip fracture: The Hordaland homocysteine study', *Journal of Bone and Mineral Research*, Vol 22(5) (2007), pp. 747–56

13 R. R. McLean, et al., 'Homocysteine as a predictive factor for hip fracture in older persons', *New England Journal of Medicine*, Vol 350(20) (2004), pp. 2042–9

14 J. B. van Meurs, et al., 'Homocysteine levels and the risk of osteoporotic fracture', *New England Journal of Medicine*, Vol 350(20) (2004), pp. 2033–41

15 M. Herrmann, et al., 'The role of hyperhomocysteinemia as well as folate, vitamin B(6) and B(12) deficiencies in osteoporosis: A systematic review', *Clinical Chemistry and Laboratory Medicine*, Vol 45(12) (2007), pp. 1621–32

16 L. G. Raisz, 'Homocysteine and osteoporotic fractures: Culprit or bystander?' *New England Journal of Medicine*, Vol 350(20) (2004), pp. 2089–90

17 G. Ravaglia, et al., 'Folate, but not homocysteine, predicts the risk of fracture in elderly persons', *The Journals of Gerontology: Series A, Biological Sciences and Medical Sciences*, Vol 60(11) (2005), pp. 1458–62; A. Cagnacci, et al., 'Relation of homocysteine, folate, and vitamin B12 to bone mineral density of postmenopausal women', *Bone*, Vol 33(6) (2003), pp. 956–9; J. Golbahar, et al., 'Association of plasma folate, plasma total homocysteine, but not methylenetetrahydrofolate reductase C667T polymorphism, with bone mineral density in postmenopausal Iranian women: A cross-sectional study', *Bone*, Vol 35(3) (2004), pp. 760–5

18 K. L. Tucker, et al., 'Low plasma vitamin B12 is associated with

lower bone mineral density: the Framingham Osteoporosis Study', *Journal of Bone and Mineral Research*, Vol 20(1) (2005), pp. 152–8; K. L. Stone, et al., 'Low serum vitamin B-12 levels are associated with increased hip bone loss in older women: A prospective study', *Journal of Clinical Endocrinology and Metabolism*, Vol 89(3) (2004), pp. 1217–21; M. S. Morris, et al., 'Relation between homocysteine and B-vitamin status indicators and bone mineral density in older Americans', *Bone*, Vol 37(2) (2005), pp. 234–42

19 R. R. McLean, et al., 'Homocysteine as a predictive factor for hip fracture in older persons', *New England Journal of Medicine*, Vol 350(20) (2004), pp. 2042–9

20 R. A. Dhonukshe-Rutten, et al., 'Vitamin B-12 status is associated with bone mineral content and bone mineral density in frail elderly women but not in men', *Journal of Nutrition*, Vol 133(3) (2003), pp. 801–7

21 R. A. Dhonukshe-Rutten, et al., 'Homocysteine and vitamin B12 status relate to bone turnover markers, broadband ultrasound attenuation, and fractures in healthy elderly people', *Journal of Bone and Mineral Research*, Vol 20(6) (2005), pp. 921–9

22 Y. Sato, et al., 'Effect of folate and mecobalamin on hip fractures in patients with stroke: A randomized controlled trial', *Journal of the American Medical Association*, Vol 293(9) (2005), pp. 1082–8

23 K. R. Dimitrova, et al., 'Estrogen and homocysteine', *Cardiovascular Research*, Vol 53(3) (2002), pp. 577–88

24 V. Mijatovic and M. J. van der Mooren, 'Homocysteine in postmenopausal women and the importance of hormone replacement therapy', *Clinical Chemistry and Laboratory Medicine*, Vol 39(8) (2001), pp. 764–7

25 G. E. Abraham, 'The importance of magnesium in the management of primary postmenopausal osteoporosis', *Journal of Nutritional Medicine*, Vol 2(2) (1991), pp. 165–78; A. R. Gaby and J. V. Wright, 'Nutrients and Osteoporosis', *Journal of Nutritional Medicine*, Vol 1(1) (1990), pp. 63–72

26 J. E. Rossouw, et al., 'Risks and benefits of estrogen plus progestin in healthy postmenopausal women: Principal results from the Women's Health Initiative randomized controlled trial', *Journal of the American Medical Association*, Vol 288(3) (2002), pp. 321–33; see also V. Beral, Million Women Study Collaborators, 'Breast cancer

and hormone-replacement therapy in the Million Women Study', *Lancet*, Vol 362(9382) (2003), pp. 419–27

27 V. Beral, Million Women Study Collaborators, 'Breast cancer and hormone-replacement therapy in the Million Women Study', *Lancet*, Vol 362(9382) (2003), pp. 419–27

28 A. Horsman, et al., 'Effect on bone of withdrawal of oestrogen therapy', *Lancet*, Vol 2(8132) (1979), p. 33

29 M. W. Tilyard, et al., 'Treatment of postmenopausal osteoporosis with calcitriol or calcium', *New England Journal of Medicine*, Vol 326(6) (1992), pp. 357–62

30 V. Matkovic, et al., 'Bone status and fracture rates in two regions of Yugoslavia', *American Journal of Clinical Nutrition*, Vol 32(3) (1979), pp. 540–9; B. E. Nordin, 'Calcium balance and calcium requirement in spinal osteoporosis', *American Journal of Clinical Nutrition*, Vol 10 (1962), pp. 384–90

31 J. C. Prior, 'Progesterone as bone-trophic hormone', *Endocrine Reviews*, Vol 11(2) (1990), pp. 386–98

32 J. C. Prior, et al., 'Spinal bone loss and ovulatory disturbances', *New England Journal of Medicine*, Vol 323(18) (1990), pp. 1221–7

33 J. R. Lee, 'Osteoporosis reversal: The role of progesterone', *International Clinical Nutrition Review*, Vol 10 (1990), pp. 384–91; J. R. Lee, 'Osteoporosis reversal with transdermal progesterone', *Lancet*, Vol 336(8726) (1990), p. 1327

34 D. Agnusdei, et al., 'A double-blind, placebo-controlled trial of ipriflavone for prevention of post-menopausal spinal bone loss', *Calcified Tissue International*, Vol 61(2) (1997), pp. 142–7; T. Ushiroyama, et al., 'Efficacy of ipriflavone and 1 alpha vitamin D therapy for the cessation of vertebral bone loss', *International Journal of Gynaecology and Obstetrics*, Vol 48(3) (1995), pp. 283–8; D. Agnusdei, et al., 'Prevention of early postmenopausal bone loss using low doses of conjugated estrogens and the non-hormonal, bone-active drug ipriflavone', *Osteoporosis International*, Vol 5(6) (1995), pp. 462–6

35 G. E. Abraham, 'The importance of magnesium in the management of primary postmenopausal osteoporosis', *Journal of Nutritional Medicine*, Vol 2(2) (1991), pp. 165–78; A. R. Gaby and J. V. Wright, 'Nutrients and osteoporosis', *Journal of Nutritional Medicine*, Vol 1(1) (1990), pp. 63–72

36 K. G. Henriksson and A. Bengtsson, 'Fibromyalgia: A clinical
    entity?' *Canadian Journal of Physiology and Pharmacology*, Vol 69(5)
    (1991), pp. 672–7

37 A. Bengtsson and K. G. Henriksson, 'The muscle in fibromyalgia –
    a review of Swedish studies', *Journal of Rheumatology*, Vol 19 (sup-
    plement) (1989), pp. 144–9

38 J. Eisinger, et al., 'Glycolysis abnormalities in fibromyalgia', *Journal
    of the American College of Nutrition*, Vol 13(2) (1994), pp. 144–8

39 M. Nicolodi and F. Sicuteri, 'Fibromyalgia and migraine. Two faces
    of the same mechanism: Serotonin as the common clue for patho-
    genesis and therapy', *Advances in Experimental Medicine and Biology*,
    Vol 398 (1996), pp. 373–9; P. Sarzi Puttini and I. Caruso, 'Primary
    fibromyalgia syndrome and 5-hydroxytryptophan: A 90-day open
    study', *Journal of International Medical Research*, Vol 20(2) (1992), pp.
    182–9. See also K. Lawson, 'Tricyclic antidepressants and
    fibromyalgia: What is the mechanism of action?', *Expert Opinion on
    Investigational Drugs*, Vol 11(10) (2002), pp. 1437–45; I. Caruso, et
    al., 'Double-blind study of 5-hydroxytryptophan versus placebo in
    the treatment of primary fibromyalgia syndrome', *Journal of Inter-
    national Medical Research*, Vol 18(3) (1990), pp. 201–9

40 M. Nicolodi and F. Sicuteri, 'Eosinophilia myalgia syndrome: The
    role of contaminants, the role of serotonergic set up', *Advances in
    Experimental Biology and Medicine*, Vol 398 (1996), pp. 351–7

41 W. B. Weglicki, et al., 'Immunoregulation by neuropeptides in
    magnesium deficiency: Ex vivo effect of enhanced substance P
    production on circulating T lymphocytes from magnesium-
    deficient mice', *Magnesium Research*, Vol 9(1) (1996), pp. 3–11

42 M. S. Seelig, 'Consequences of magnesium deficiency on the
    enhancement of stress reactions: Preventive and therapeutic impli-
    cations (a review)', *Journal of the American College of Nutrition*, Vol
    13(5) (1994), pp. 429–46

43 G. E. Abraham and J. Flechas, 'Management of fibromyalgia:
    Rational for the use of magnesium and malic acid', *Journal of
    Nutritional Medicine*, Vol 3 (1992), pp. 49–59; V. Bobyleva-Guarriero
    and H. A. Lardy, 'The role of malate in exercise-induced enhance-
    ment of mitochondrial respiration', *Archives of Biochemistry and
    Biophysics*, Vol 245(2) (1986), pp. 470–6

44 M. F. Holick, 'Vitamin D: importance in the prevention of cancers,

type 1 diabetes, heart disease, and osteoporosis', *American Journal of Clinical Nutrition*, Vol 79(3) (2004), pp. 362–71

45 B. Regland, et al., 'Increased concentrations of homocysteine in the cerebrospinal fluid in patients with fibromyalgia and chronic fatigue syndrome', *Scandinavian Journal of Rheumatology*, Vol 26(4) (1997), pp. 301–7

46 G. A. Tate, et al., 'Suppression of monosodium urate crystal-induced acute inflammation by diets enriched with gamma-linolenic acid and eicosapentaenoic acid', *Arthritis and Rheumatism*, Vol 31(12) (1988), pp. 1543–51

47 R. A. Jacob, et al., 'Consumption of cherries lowers plasma urate in healthy women', *Journal of Nutrition*, Vol 133(6) (2003), pp. 1826–9

48 H. Wang, et al., 'Antioxidant and anti-inflammatory activities of anthocyanins and their aglycon, cyanidin, from tart cherries', *Journal of Natural Products*, Vol 62(2) (1999), pp. 294–6; N. P. Seeram, et al., 'Cyclooxygenase inhibitory and antioxidant cyanidin glycosides in cherries and berries', *Phytomedicine*, Vol 8(5) (2001), pp. 362–9; N. P. Seeram, et al., 'Degradation products of cyanidin glycosides from tart cherries and their bioactivities', *Journal of Agricultural and Food Chemistry*, Vol 49(10) (2001), pp. 4924–9; J. M. Tall, et al., 'Tart cherry anthocyanins suppress inflammation-induced pain behavior in rat', *Behavioural Brain Research*, Vol 153(1) (2004), pp. 181–8

Part 5

1 S. Davies, 'Nutritional Flat Earthers' (Editorial), *Journal of Nutritional Medicine*, Vol 1(3) (1990), pp. 167–70

2 MAAF, *Household Food Consumption and Expenditure*, HMSO (1991)

3 Booker Health Report (1985)

4 NACNE, 'Proposals for nutritional guidelines for health education in Britain', Health Education Council (1983)

5 A. Vogiatzoglou, et al., 'Vitamin B12 status and rate of brain volume loss in community-dwelling elderly', *Neurology*, Vol 71(11) (2008), pp. 826–32

6 RSC Food Chemistry Symposium (November 1992)

7 RSC Food Chemistry Symposium (November 1992)

8 RSC Food Chemistry Symposium (November 1992)

9   *The Vitamin Controversy*, ION (1987)

10   F. R. Ellis, et al., 'Incidence of osteoporosis in vegetarians and omnivores', *American Journal of Clinical Nutrition*, Vol 25(6) (1972), pp. 555–8

11   A. G. Marsh, et al., 'Cortical bone density of adult lacto-ovo-vegetarian and omnivorous women', *Journal of the American Dietetic Association*, Vol 76(2) (1980), pp. 148–51

12   Lucas and Power, *Clinical Research*, Vol 29(4), (1981), p. 754

13   L. Skoldstam, 'Fasting and vegan diet in rheumatoid arthritis', *Scandinavian Journal of Rheumatology*, Vol 15(2) (1986), pp. 219–21

14   M. Gabor, 'Pharmacologic effects of flavonoids on blood vessels', *Angiologica*, Vol 9(3–6) (1972), pp. 355–74; J. Kuhnau, 'The flavonoids. A class of semi-essential food components: their role in human nutrition', *World Review of Nutrition and Dietetics*, Vol 24 (1976), pp. 117–91; B. Havsteen, 'Flavonoids, a class of natural products of high pharmacological potency', *Biochemical Pharmacology*, Vol 32(7) (1983), pp. 1141–8; E. Middleton Jr and C. Kandaswami, 'Effects of flavonoids on immune and inflammatory cell functions', *Biochemical Pharmacology*, Vol 43(6) (1992), pp. 1167–79

15   Neligan and Salt, *Lancet*, Vol 2 (1934), p. 209

16   A. E. Osterberg, et al., 'The absorption of sulphur compounds during treatment by sulphur baths', *Archives of Dermatology and Syphilology*, Vol 20(2) (1929), pp. 158–66

17   A. J. Hartz, et al., 'The association of obesity with joint pain and osteoarthritis in the HANES data', *Journal of Chronic Diseases*, Vol 39(4) (1986), pp. 311–19

18   R. M. Acheson and A. B. Collart, 'New Haven survey of joint diseases. XVII: Relationship between some systemic characteristics and osteoarthrosis in a general population', *Annals of the Rheumatic Diseases*, Vol 34(5) (1975), pp. 379–87; J. S. Lawrence, 'Hypertension in relation to musculoskeletal disorders', *Annals of the Rheumatic Diseases*, Vol 34(5) (1975), pp. 451–6

19   W. Solomon on J. Bland, Nutrition Symposium tape (1984)

20   E. L. Smith Jr., et al., 'Physical activity and calcium modalities for bone mineral increase in aged women', *Medicine and Science in Sports and Exercise*, Vol 13(1) (1981), pp. 60–4

21   *New Scientist* (15/8/92)

Recommended Reading

Darlington, Dr G. and Gamlin, L., *Diet and Arthritis*, Vermilion (1998)

Friedberger, J., *Office Yoga*, Motilal Banarsidass (1999)

Germano, C. with Cabot, W., *The Osteoporosis Solution*, Kensington Publishing (1999)

Holford, P. and Braly, Dr J., *Hidden Food Allergies*, Piatkus (2005)

Holford, P. and Braly, Dr J., *The H Factor*, Piatkus (2003)

Holford, P. and Burne, J., *Food is Better Medicine Than Drugs*, Piatkus (2006)

Holford, P. and McDonald Joyce, F., *Food GLorious Food*, Piatkus (2008)

Holford, P. and McDonald Joyce, F., *The Holford 9-Day Liver Detox*, Piatkus (2007)

Holford, P. and McDonald Joyce, F., *The Holford Low-GL Diet Cookbook*, Piatkus (2005)

Holford, P. and Ridgway, J., *The Optimum Nutrition Cookbook*, Piatkus (2000)

Holford, P., *The Holford Low-GL Diet Made Easy*, Piatkus (2007)

Holford, P., *The Low-GL Diet Bible*, Piatkus (2009)

Holford, P., *Beat Stress and Fatigue*, Piatkus (1999)

Holford, P., *Improve Your Digestion and Absorption*, Piatkus (1999)

Holford, P., *The New Optimum Nutrition Bible*, Piatkus (2004)

Jacob, S.W., MD, Lawrence, R.M., MD, PhD and Zucker, M., *The Miracle of MSM: The Natural Solution For Pain*, G P Putnam's Sons (1999)

Sayce, V. and Fraser, I., *Exercise Beats Arthritis*, Thorsons (1999)

RESOURCES

The Holford Diet Club, called Zest4Life, is based on low GL principles and provides advice and support for weight loss through a series of weekly meetings. For more information, visit www.zest4life.eu.

The Institute for Optimum Nutrition (ION) offers a three-year foundation degree course in nutritional therapy that includes training in the optimum nutrition approach to mental health. There is a clinic, a list of nutrition practitioners across the UK, an information service and a quarterly journal, *Optimum Nutrition*. Visit www.ion.ac.uk, address: Avalon House, 72 Lower Mortlake Road, Richmond, TW9 2JY, UK, tel: +44 (0)870 979 1122.

Nutritional therapy and consultations To find a nutritional therapist near you who I would recommend, visit www.patrickholford.com. This service gives details on who to see in the UK as well as internationally. If there is no one available nearby, you can always take an on-line assessment – see below.

Naturopaths To find a registered naturopath near you, contact The General Council and Register of Naturopaths at

Goswell House, 2 Goswell Road, Street, BA16 0JG, tel: +44 (0)8707 456984 or visit: www.naturopathy.org.uk and search under 'find a member'.

On-line 100% Health Programme How 100 per cent healthy are you? Find out with our FREE health check and comprehensive personalised 100% Health Programme, giving you a personalised action plan, including diet and supplements. Visit www.patrickholford.com.

Water filters There are many water filters on the market. One of the best is offered by The Fresh Water Filter Company, who produce mains-attached water-filtering units using gravity rather than reverse osmosis (which can filter out some useful minerals as well). You can buy a whole-house filter or an under-sink version. Visit www.freshwaterfilter.com.

Psychocalisthenics is an excellent exercise system that takes less than 20 minutes a day, and develops strength, suppleness and stamina as well as generating vital energy. The best way to learn it is to do the Psychocalisthenics Training. See www.patrickholdford.com (events) for details on this. Also available is the book *Master Level Exercise: Psychocalisthenics*, and the Psychocalisthenics CD and DVD, available from www.patrickholford.com. For further information please see www.pcals.com.

Arthritis Care has a 43-page downloadable pdf called *Exercise and Arthritis* with specific exercises such as range of motion, strengthening exercises, and so on. See www.arthritiscare.org.uk.

General Osteopathic Council For information, or to find an osteopath in your area, visit www.osteopathy.org.uk, tel: +44 (0)20 7357 6655 or write to: General Osteopathic Council, 176 Tower Bridge Road, London SE1 3LU.

Clive Lathey's osteopathic practice (Clive Lathey contributed to Chapter 24), is in Putney, London. Visit www. putneyclinic.co.uk, tel: +44 (0)20 8789 3881.

General Chiropractic Council For information, or to find a chiropractor in your area, visit www.gcc-uk.org, tel: + 44 (0)20 7713 5155 or write to: General Chiropractic Council, 44 Wicklow Street, London, WC1X 9HL.

Alexander Technique The Society of Teachers of the Alexander Technique (STAT), 20 London House, 266 Fulham Road, London SW10 9EL. Tel: +44 (0)20 7351 0828. They will send you a free directory – write with a stamped addressed envelope.

The Back Shop specialises in Back Care Solutions, providing a variety of products for the home, office and car, including chairs, and fitness and posture aids. They have a showroom at 14 New Cavendish Street, London, W1G 8UW. Visit www.thebackshop.co.uk, or tel: +44 (0)20 7935 9120/9148.

Klass Vaki is a contoured mattress that goes on your bed and dramatically reduces pressure on bones and joints. Available from Totally Nourish (see below).

The Natural Progesterone Information Service (NPIS) provides women and their doctors with information on natural progesterone and details of how to obtain natural progesterone information packs, as well as books relating to natural hormone health. Visit www.npis.info/ for more information; tel: 07000 784849, address: NPIS, PO Box 24, Buxton, SK17 9FB.

Salt alternatives The average person gets far too much sodium because we eat too much salt (sodium chloride) and salted foods, and not enough potassium and magnesium, found in fruits and vegetables. The net result is water retention and weight gain, anxiety, insomnia, high blood pressure and muscle cramps. Not all salt, however, is bad for you. Solo Low Sodium Sea Salt contains 60 per cent less sodium and is high in the essential minerals of magnesium and potassium. Available from health-food stores and supermarkets. Their 200g (7oz) reusable shaker is sold in the UK, Ireland, Spain, the Netherlands, Singapore, Hong Kong, Japan, Bahrain, Saudi Arabia, the United Arab Emirates, Jordon, the Baltic States and the United States of America. Visit their website: www.soloseasalt.com for more information or call their international help line on: +44 845 130 4568, or 020 8464 1665 if you are in the UK.

Sugar alternative Xylitol is a low GL natural sugar alternative, available from high-street health-food stores. Also available by mail order from Totally Nourish (see below), sold as XyloBrit.

CherryActive is sold in a highly concentrated juice format. Mix a 30ml (1fl oz) serving with 250ml (9fl oz) water to make a deliciously healthy, low-GL cherry juice. Each 946ml bottle contains the juice from over 3,000 cherries – that's half a tree's worth – and contains a month's supply. CherryActive is also available as a dried cherry snack and in capsules. For more information and to order, visit Totally Nourish (see p. 353).

LABORATORY TESTS

Food allergy (IgG ELISA), homocysteine and liver-check tests are available through YorkTest Laboratories, using a home-test kit where you can take your own pinprick blood sample and return it to the lab for analysis. Visit www.yorktest.com, address: Freepost, NEA5 243, York, YO19 5ZZ, tel: freephone (in UK) 0800 0746185. Also see www.thehfactor.com for details of other labs and what to supplement, depending on your results.

Intestinal permeability (leaky gut) test This test is available from the following labs through qualified nutrition consultants and doctors:
Biolab Medical Unit (doctor's referral only): visit www.biolab.co.uk or call +44 (0)20 7636 5959/5905.
Genova Diagnostics (formerly Individual Wellbeing Diagnostic Laboratory): visit www.gdx.uk.net or call +44 (0)20 8336 7750.

Hair mineral analyses, to determine the presence of any toxic metals, can be arranged via your local nutritional therapist (see www.patrickholford.com for a referral) or are available from Mineral Check, tel: +44 (0) 1622 850500, or visit www.mineralcheck.com. Also available from Totally Nourish (see p. 353).

SUPPLEMENT, REMEDY AND SUPPLIER DIRECTORY

Finding your own perfect supplement programme can be confusing, but my website, www.patrickholford.com, offers useful guidance. The backbone of a good supplement programme is:

- A high-strength multivitamin.
- Additional vitamin C.
- An essential fat supplement containing omega-3 and omega-6 oils.

In this section are examples of supplements that provide the herbs and nutrients at the levels discussed in this book. The addresses of the companies whose products I've referred to are given at the end.

Antioxidants

A good all-round antioxidant complex should provide vitamin A (beta-carotene and/or retinol), vitamins C and E, zinc, selenium, glutathione or cysteine, anthocyanidins of berry extracts, lipoic acid and co-enzyme Q_{10}. See BioCare's AGE Antioxidant followed by Solgar's Advanced Antioxidant Nutrients. Complexes of bioflavonoids, often found together with vitamin C, are available from both companies.

Bone health

Minerals such as calcium, magnesium, boron, zinc and silica plus vitamin C and D all help support bone health. Try Solgar's Advanced Calcium Complex and BioCare's Osteoplex.

Digestive enzymes and support

Any decent digestive enzyme needs to contain enzymes to digest protein (protease), carbohydrate (amylase) and fat (lipase). Some also contain amyloglucosidase, which digests glucosides found in certain beans and vegetables noted for their flatulent effects. Try Solgar's Vegan Digestive Enzymes. BioCare's DigestPro contains these enzymes and probiotics.

Some people have low levels of betaine hydrochloride (stomach acid). You can supplement this on its own and, if it helps digestion, this might be your problem. Solgar's Digestive Aid supplement contains betaine HCL, plus other digestive enzymes. It is not vegetarian.

Essential fats and fish oil supplements

The most important omega-3 fats are DHA and EPA, the richest source being cod liver oil. The most important omega-6 fat is GLA, the richest source being borage (also known as starflower) oil. Try BioCare's Essential Omegas, which provides a highly concentrated mix of EPA, DHA and GLA. They also produce Mega-EPA, a high potency omega-3 fish oil supplement. Also, Seven Seas Extra High Strength Cod Liver Oil. Both these products have consistently proven the purest when tested for PCB residues, which are in almost all fish. Cod liver oil also contains vitamin A. BioCare's Mega GLA Complex and Solgar's One-A-Day GLA are good value if you only want omega-6 fats.

Homocysteine modulators containing TMG (trimethylglycine)

BioCare's Connect. Ingredients include TMG, vitamin B_6, riboflavin (vitamin B_2), zinc, folic acid and vitamin B_{12}.

Solgar's Gold Specifics Homocysteine Modulators. Ingredients include TMG, vitamin B_6, vitamin B_{12}, and folic acid.

Higher Nature's 'H Factors'. Ingredients include vitamin B_{12} and zinc.

Joint-support supplements and balms

Look for combinations of boswellia, curcumin, hop extract, olive extract, glucosamine and MSM. Best taken with omega-3 fish oils.

BioCare's Joint Support is a potent combination of amino acids and botanicals to support healthy joints. Glucosamine hydrochloride and MSM provide structural support to the joints, while MSM combines with hops, olive extract, curcumin and quercetin to maintain healthy joints.

Solgar's Gold Specifics Joint Modulators include glucosamine sulfate, DLPA (DL-phenylalanine), standardised turmeric powdered extract, vitamin C, niacin (as niacinamide) and manganese.

Arnica: the arnica gel used in a study quoted on page 55 was A. Vogel Arnica Gel, sold as Bioforce A. Vogel Atrogel Arnica Gel. Look for it in health-food stores or order online.

Others: look for creams or gels containing any, or a combination of the nutrients or herbs discussed in Chapter 5. Examples include Optima Musseltone Gel – Green Lipped Mussel Extract with Glucosamine and Nature's Plus Glucosamine Chondroitin MSM with Celadrin and Black Cherry Cream – available online or from independent health-food stores.

Celadrin (also available in capsules) is available from Solgar (see below), independent health-food stores and online.

Multivitamin and mineral supplements

Supplementing the right multivitamin is the most important supplement decision you make. Most multis are based on RDA levels of nutrients, which are not the same as optimum-nutrition levels. The best multivitamin based on optimum-nutrition levels, is BioCare's Advanced Optimum Nutrition Formula. The second best is Solgar's VM2000. Both of these recommend taking two tablets a day. Advanced Optimum Nutrition Formula has better mineral levels, especially for calcium and magnesium. Ideally, both should be taken with an extra 1g of vitamin C.

Probiotics

Probiotics are supplements of beneficial bacteria, the two main strains being *Lactobacillus acidophilus* and *Bifidobacterium bifidus*. There are various types of strains within these two, some more important in children, others in adults. There is quite some variability in amounts of bacteria (some labels say things like 'a billion viable organisms per capsule') and quality. A very good product is BioCare's Bio-Acidophilus and also Digestpro, which also contains digestive enzymes.

SAMe (s-adenosyl methionine) is currently unavailable in the UK. However, Nature Made (www.naturemade.com) produce a high-quality SAMe product called Mood Plus, which is available in the US. SAMe is also available in South Africa.

SUPPLEMENT RESOURCES

The following companies produce good-quality supplements that are widely available in the UK.

BioCare offers an extensive range of nutritional and herbal supplements, including daily 'packs'. Their products are stocked by most good health-food shops. Visit www.biocare.co.uk, tel: +44 (0)121 433 3727. They are also available by mail order from Totally Nourish (www.totally nourish.com) – see opposite.

Totally Nourish is the best 'e'-health shop that stocks many high-quality health products, including home-test kits, Get Up & Go (the low-GL powdered breakfast drink referred to in Chapter 22) and supplements. Visit www.totallynourish.com, tel: 0800 085 7749 (freephone within the UK). Outside the UK, tel: +44 (0)20 8788 9242, address: Lakeside, 180 Lifford Lane, Kings Norton, Birmingham, B30 3NU.

Seven Seas specialise in cod liver oil, rich in omega-3 fats. Available in health-food stores and pharmacies. Website: www.seven-seas.ltd.uk

Solgar products are available in most independent health-food stores or visit www.solgar-vitamins.co.uk, tel: +44 (0) 1442 890355.

And in other regions:

South Africa

Bioharmony produce a wide range of products in South Africa and other African countries. For details of your nearest supplier visit www.bioharmony.co.za, tel: 0860 888 339.

Australia

Solgar supplements are available in Australia. Visit www.solgar.com.au, tel: 1800 029 871 (free call) for your nearest supplier. Another good brand is Blackmores.

New Zealand

BioCare products (see above) are available in New Zealand through Aurora Natural Therapies. Visit www.Aurora.org.nz, address: 12a Battys Road, Springlands, Blenheim 7201, New Zealand.

Singapore

BioCare (see above) and **Solgar** products are available in Singapore through Essential Living. Visit www.essliv.com, tel: 6276 1380.

UAE

BioCare supplements (see above) are available in Dubai from Nutripharm FZCO, address: Post Box: 71246, Dubai, United Arab Emirates, tel: +971–4-3410008, fax: +971–4-3410009.

INDEX

Note: Page numbers in **bold** refer to illustrations.

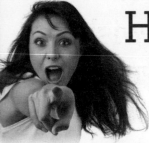

How 100% Healthy are you?

"I thought I was a healthy person. I did the online report. I feel absolutely fantastic. It's changed my life. It's amazing." Karen S

Karen before
36%

Karen after
86%

D	C	B	A
NOT GOOD	AVERAGE	REASONABLY HEALTHY	HEALTHY

YOU CAN wake up full of energy, with a clear mind and balanced mood, never gain weight and stay disease free. Having worked with over 60,000 people We know what changes are going to most rapidly transform how you feel. The **100% Health Programme** is the most comprehensive and genuinely effective way of taking a step towards 100% health.

Your **FREE Health Check** is the first step to receiving your **100% Health Programme** (£24.95), the ultimate on-line personal health profile, that shows you exactly what your perfect diet and daily supplement programme is, and which simple lifestyle changes will make the biggest difference.

You receive:

✔ A full Set of Results on your body systems and processes

✔ In-depth Report on you & your health

✔ Your Perfect Recipes and Menu Plan

✔ Your own Library of Special Reports

✔ Full Lifestyle Analysis inc:
  • Exercise • Stress • Sleep • Pollution

✔ Your Action Plan & Personal Supplement Programme;

✔ PLUS optional weekly support and guidance from Patrick;

✔ Free Reassessment to chart your progress, month by month

✔ Your questions answered by Patrick himself, plus all the benefits of membership

BEGIN YOUR **FREE** HEALTH CHECKUP NOW
Go to **www.patrickholford.com**

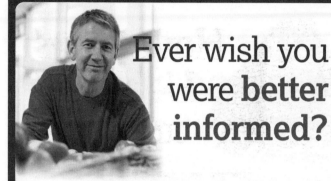

100%Health®
Weekend Intensive
The workshop that works.